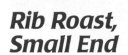

Rib Roast, Small End
(Prime Rib Premium Oven Roast)

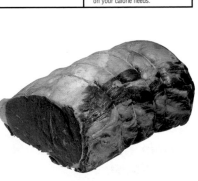

- Roast in a preheated 350°F (177°C) oven to an internal temperature of 145°F (63°C) for medium rare; 155°F (68°C) for medium. Let roast rest 15 to 20 minutes before carving.

Tip: This 3-rib roast is the small end of the ribs adjacent to the short loin. It is next to the T-bone, porterhouse grilling, New York strip and tenderloin area. Rib roast is best cooked to the rare side.

Nutrition Facts	Amount Per 3-Ounce (85-Gram) Serving, (cooked)			
Calories	360	Total Carbohydrate* 0g 0%	Vitamin A*	0%
Calories from Fat 280		Dietary Fiber* 0g 0%	Vitamin C*	0%
Total Fat*	31g 45%	Sugars 0g	Calcium*	0%
Saturated Fat*	13g 70%	Protein 19g	Iron*	10%
Cholesterol*	70mg 25%	Potassium 269mg	* Percent Daily Values are based on a 2,000 calorie diet. Your daily values may be higher or lower, depending on your calorie needs.	
Sodium*	55mg 2%			

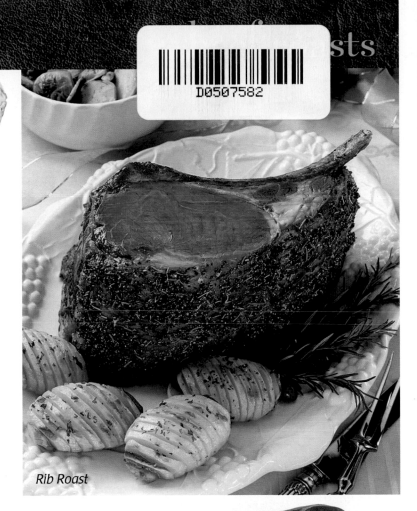

Rib Roast

Rib Roast, Large End
(Standing Rib Premium Oven Roast)

- Roast in a preheated 350°F (177°C) oven until internal temperature is 145°F (63°C) for medium rare; 155°F (68°C) for medium. A 6- to 8-pound (2.73 to 3.64kg) roast cooks about 2½ hours. Let roast rest 15 to 20 minutes.

Tip: The large end of the rib is tender and flavorful. Ask the butcher to trim off the chine bone to make carving easier.

Nutrition Facts	Amount Per 3-Ounce (85-Gram) Serving, (cooked)			
Calories	350	Total Carbohydrate* 0g 0%	Vitamin A*	0%
Calories from Fat 270		Dietary Fiber* 0g 0%	Vitamin C*	0%
Total Fat*	29g 45%	Sugars 0g	Calcium*	0%
Saturated Fat*	12g 60%	Protein 19g	Iron*	10%
Cholesterol*	70mg 25%	Potassium 240mg	* Percent Daily Values are based on a 2,000 calorie diet. Your daily values may be higher or lower, depending on your calorie needs.	
Sodium*	55mg 2%			

Cross Rib Roast
(Cross Rib Pot Roast)

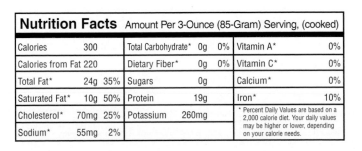

- Brown roast on all sides. Place in a heavy, lidded casserole. Add ½ to 2 cups (118 to 473ml) broth, water or wine. Cover and cook in preheated 325°F (163°C) oven 2 to 3 hours, depending on size, or until meat is tender.

Tip: Pieces of the chuck are boneless flat roasts or rolled and tied. All chuck cuts such as the cross rib roast make excellent pot roasts. This roast has good texture and rich, beefy flavor.

Nutrition Facts	Amount Per 3-Ounce (85-Gram) Serving, (cooked)			
Calories	300	Total Carbohydrate* 0g 0%	Vitamin A*	0%
Calories from Fat 220		Dietary Fiber* 0g 0%	Vitamin C*	0%
Total Fat*	24g 35%	Sugars 0g	Calcium*	0%
Saturated Fat*	10g 50%	Protein 19g	Iron*	10%
Cholesterol*	70mg 25%	Potassium 260mg	* Percent Daily Values are based on a 2,000 calorie diet. Your daily values may be higher or lower, depending on your calorie needs.	
Sodium*	55mg 2%			

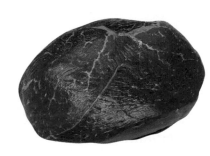

Rib Eye Roast, Boneless
(Rib Eye Premium Oven Roast)

- Roast in preheated 350°F (177°C) oven to an internal temperature of 145°F (63°C) for medium rare; 155°F (68°C) for medium. Let roast rest 15 to 20 minutes before carving.

Tip: One of the most flavorful boneless roasts, it is a delicious roast with little waste that can be cut to any size for roasting or sliced for steaks.

Nutrition Facts		Amount Per 3-Ounce (85-Gram) Serving, (cooked)				
Calories	260	Total Carbohydrate*	0g	0%	Vitamin A*	0%
Calories from Fat 170		Dietary Fiber*	0g	0%	Vitamin C*	0%
Total Fat*	19g 30%	Sugars		0g	Calcium*	0%
Saturated Fat*	8g 40%	Protein		21g	Iron*	10%
Cholesterol*	70mg 25%	Potassium		292mg	* Percent Daily Values are based on a 2,000 calorie diet. Your daily values may be higher or lower, depending on your calorie needs.	
Sodium*	55mg 2%					

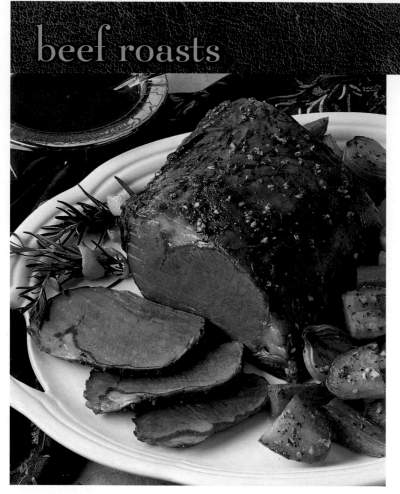

Rib Eye Roast

Rib Eye Roast, Bone-In
(Prime Rib Oven Roast)

- Roast in preheated 350°F (177°C) oven to an internal temperature of 145°F (63°C) for medium rare; 155°F (68°C) for medium. Let roast rest 15 to 20 minutes before carving.

Tip: This roast has rib bones attached, but fat and chine bones removed for easy carving. A 5-rib roast serves 10. A rolled roast requires 5 to 10 more minutes per pound (.45kg).

Nutrition Facts		Amount Per 3-Ounce (85-Gram) Serving, (cooked)				
Calories	260	Total Carbohydrate*	0g	0%	Vitamin A*	0%
Calories from Fat 170		Dietary Fiber*	0g	0%	Vitamin C*	0%
Total Fat*	19g 30%	Sugars		0g	Calcium*	0%
Saturated Fat*	8g 40%	Protein		21g	Iron*	10%
Cholesterol*	70mg 25%	Potassium		292mg	* Percent Daily Values are based on a 2,000 calorie diet. Your daily values may be higher or lower, depending on your calorie needs.	
Sodium*	55mg 2%					

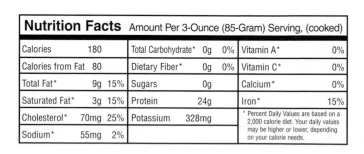

Sirloin Tip Roast
(Sirloin Tip Oven Roast)

- Roast in preheated 350°F (177°C) oven to an internal temperature of 145°F (63°C) for medium rare; 155°F (68°C) for medium. Let roast rest 15 to 20 minutes before carving.

Tip: Less expensive, it has little waste and tastes great with proper preparation. Use a dry rub or wet marinade for added flavor.

Nutrition Facts		Amount Per 3-Ounce (85-Gram) Serving, (cooked)				
Calories	180	Total Carbohydrate*	0g	0%	Vitamin A*	0%
Calories from Fat 80		Dietary Fiber*	0g	0%	Vitamin C*	0%
Total Fat*	9g 15%	Sugars		0g	Calcium*	0%
Saturated Fat*	3g 15%	Protein		24g	Iron*	15%
Cholesterol*	70mg 25%	Potassium		328mg	* Percent Daily Values are based on a 2,000 calorie diet. Your daily values may be higher or lower, depending on your calorie needs.	
Sodium*	55mg 2%					

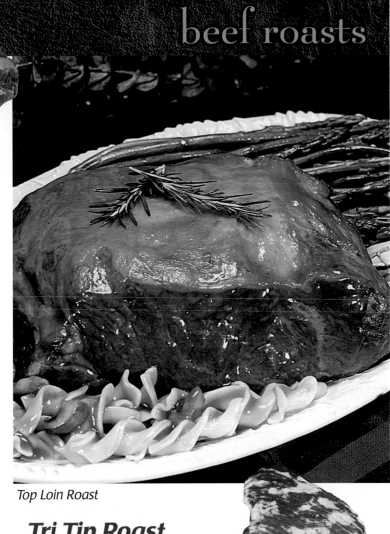

Top Loin Roast
(Strip Loin Premium Oven Roast)

- Roast in preheated 350°F (177°C) oven to an internal temperature of 145°F (63°C) for medium rare; 155°F (68°C) for medium. Let roast rest 15 to 20 minutes before carving.

Tip: This flavorful, tender roast is from the short loin area. It can be roasted whole to serve a crowd. Carve into ½-inch (1.27cm) thick slices.

Nutrition Facts	Amount Per 3-Ounce (85-Gram) Serving, (cooked)			
Calories 250	Total Carbohydrate* 0g 0%		Vitamin A*	0%
Calories from Fat 160	Dietary Fiber* 0g 0%		Vitamin C*	0%
Total Fat* 18g 25%	Sugars 0g		Calcium*	0%
Saturated Fat* 7g 35%	Protein 22g		Iron*	10%
Cholesterol* 65mg 20%	Potassium 295mg		* Percent Daily Values are based on a 2,000 calorie diet. Your daily values may be higher or lower, depending on your calorie needs.	
Sodium* 55mg 2%				

Top Loin Roast

Tenderloin Roast
(Tenderloin Premium Oven Roast)

- Roast a 2- to 3-pound (.91 to 1.36kg) tenderloin in a preheated 425°F (218°C) oven 35 to 40 minutes for medium rare; a 4- to 5-pound (1.82 to 2.27kg) tenderloin roasts 50 to 60 minutes for medium rare. Add 10 minutes for medium. Let roast rest 15 to 20 minutes before carving.

Tip: This roast is sold whole or in sections. It is the easiest and quickest cut to roast – full of flavor and very tender.

Tri Tip Roast
(Bottom Sirloin Tri Tip Oven Roast)

- Roast a 1½- to 2-pound (.68 to .91kg) tri tip roast in preheated 425°F (218°C) oven 30 to 40 minutes for medium rare. Add 5 to 10 minutes for medium. Let roast rest 15 to 20 minutes before carving.

Tip: Tri tip is lean, tender, and full-flavored – a great value. Pastes, made with a variety of herbs and spices, can be rubbed over the roast, creating a luscious crust when cooked.

Nutrition Facts	Amount Per 3-Ounce (85-Gram) Serving, (cooked)			
Calories 200	Total Carbohydrate* 0g 0%		Vitamin A*	0%
Calories from Fat 100	Dietary Fiber* 0g 0%		Vitamin C*	0%
Total Fat* 11g 15%	Sugars 0g		Calcium*	0%
Saturated Fat* 4g 20%	Protein 24g		Iron*	15%
Cholesterol* 70mg 25%	Potassium 356mg		* Percent Daily Values are based on a 2,000 calorie diet. Your daily values may be higher or lower, depending on your calorie needs.	
Sodium* 55mg 2%				

Nutrition Facts	Amount Per 3-Ounce (85-Gram) Serving, (cooked)			
Calories 210	Total Carbohydrate* 0g 0%		Vitamin A*	0%
Calories from Fat 100	Dietary Fiber* 0g 0%		Vitamin C*	0%
Total Fat* 11g 17%	Sugars 0g		Calcium*	2%
Saturated Fat* 4g 20%	Protein 26g		Iron*	20%
Cholesterol* 55mg 18%	Potassium 385mg		* Percent Daily Values are based on a 2,000 calorie diet. Your daily values may be higher or lower, depending on your calorie needs.	
Sodium* 60mg 3%				

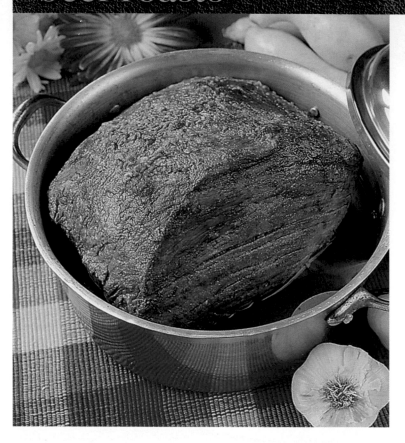

Eye of Round Roast
(Eye of Round Oven Roast)

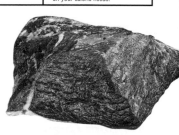

- Roast an eye of round roast in preheated 325°F (163°C) oven for 1½ to 1¾ hours for medium rare. Add 15 minutes for medium. Let roast rest 15 to 20 minutes before carving. For added flavor, first marinate in garlic, fresh basil leaves and olive oil. Slice thinly.

Tip: This oven roast is lean and boneless with little fat. Marinating in vinegar, wine and spices improves both flavor and texture.

Nutrition Facts	Amount Per 3-Ounce (85-Gram) Serving, (cooked)				
Calories	160	Total Carbohydrate*	0g 0%	Vitamin A*	0%
Calories from Fat 60		Dietary Fiber*	0g 0%	Vitamin C*	0%
Total Fat*	6g 10%	Sugars	0g	Calcium*	0%
Saturated Fat*	2.5g 10%	Protein	24g	Iron*	10%
Cholesterol*	60mg 20%	Potassium	324mg	* Percent Daily Values are based on a 2,000 calorie diet. Your daily values may be higher or lower, depending on your calorie needs.	
Sodium*	50mg 2%				

Round Rump Roast

Round Rump Roast
(Round Rump Oven Roast)

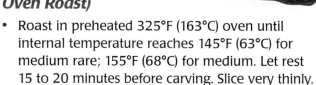

- Brown slowly on all sides. Add ½ to 2 cups (118 to 473ml) broth, water, juice, wine or beer. Bring to boil. Cover and roast in preheated 325°F (163°C) oven for 2¾ to 3¼ hours. Let roast rest 15 to 20 minutes before carving. Slice thinly.

Tip: Thawing frozen roasts in the refrigerator isn't just a safe choice, it's a smart one. In the refrigerator, ice crystals melt slowly so they're reabsorbed into the meat, adding juiciness.

Nutrition Facts	Amount Per 3-Ounce (85-Gram) Serving, (cooked)				
Calories	240	Total Carbohydrate*	0g 0%	Vitamin A*	0%
Calories from Fat 140		Dietary Fiber*	0g 0%	Vitamin C*	0%
Total Fat*	15g 23%	Sugars	0g	Calcium*	0%
Saturated Fat*	6g 30%	Protein	24g	Iron*	15%
Cholesterol*	80mg 27%	Potassium	240mg	* Percent Daily Values are based on a 2,000 calorie diet. Your daily values may be higher or lower, depending on your calorie needs.	
Sodium*	45mg 2%				

Bottom Round Roast
(Outside Round Oven Roast)

- Roast in preheated 325°F (163°C) oven until internal temperature reaches 145°F (63°C) for medium rare; 155°F (68°C) for medium. Let rest 15 to 20 minutes before carving. Slice very thinly.
- Braise at 325°F (163°C) in ½ to 2 cups (118 to 473ml) liquid. A 3-pound (1.36kg) roast cooks 3 hours.

Tip: Traditionally, bottom round roast is used to make sauerbraten. It is a boneless muscle from the back leg with little fat.

Nutrition Facts	Amount Per 3-Ounce (85-Gram) Serving, (cooked)				
Calories	180	Total Carbohydrate*	0g 0%	Vitamin A*	0%
Calories from Fat 70		Dietary Fiber*	0g 0%	Vitamin C*	0%
Total Fat*	7g 10%	Sugars	0g	Calcium*	0%
Saturated Fat*	2.5g 10%	Protein	27g	Iron*	15%
Cholesterol*	80mg 25%	Potassium	262mg	* Percent Daily Values are based on a 2,000 calorie diet. Your daily values may be higher or lower, depending on your calorie needs.	
Sodium*	45mg 0%				

Top Round Roast
(Inside Round Roast)

- Roast a top round roast in preheated 325°F (163°C) oven to an internal temperature of 145°F (63°C) for medium rare; 155°F (68°C) for medium. This meat is best cooked slowly at a low temperature. Take care to keep the meat moist. Let roast rest 15 to 20 minutes.

Tip: Top round has good flavor, texture and juiciness. It is often used for roast beef sandwiches.

Nutrition Facts		Amount Per 3-Ounce (85-Gram) Serving, (cooked)			
Calories	160	Total Carbohydrate*	0g 0%	Vitamin A*	0%
Calories from Fat 30		Dietary Fiber*	0g 0%	Vitamin C*	0%
Total Fat*	3.5g 6%	Sugars	0g	Calcium*	0%
Saturated Fat*	1g 6%	Protein	31g	Iron*	15%
Cholesterol*	75mg 25%	Potassium	284mg	* Percent Daily Values are based on a 2,000 calorie diet. Your daily values may be higher or lower, depending on your calorie needs.	
Sodium*	40mg 0%				

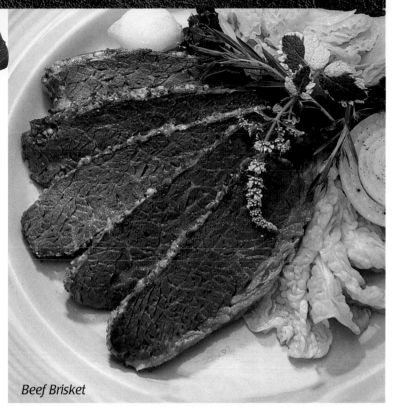

Beef Brisket

Chuck Roast, Boneless
(Blade Pot Roast)

- Brown on all sides. Place in a heavy, lidded casserole. Add ½ to 2 cups (118 to 473ml) broth, water or wine. Cover and cook in a preheated 325°F (163°C) oven for 2 to 3 hours or until meat is fork-tender.

Tip: Meat from the chuck is always an excellent choice for pot roast. A pot roast can be cooked in advance. Just add vegetables and thicken broth right before serving.

Nutrition Facts		Amount Per 3-Ounce (85-Gram) Serving, (cooked)			
Calories	200	Total Carbohydrate*	0g 0%	Vitamin A*	0%
Calories from Fat 90		Dietary Fiber*	0g 0%	Vitamin C*	0%
Total Fat*	10g 15%	Sugars	0g	Calcium*	0%
Saturated Fat*	4g 20%	Protein	26g	Iron*	15%
Cholesterol*	90mg 30%	Potassium	224mg	* Percent Daily Values are based on a 2,000 calorie diet. Your daily values may be higher or lower, depending on your calorie needs.	
Sodium*	60mg 2%				

Brisket, Boneless
(Brisket Pot Roast)

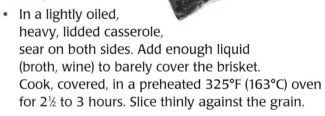

- In a lightly oiled, heavy, lidded casserole, sear on both sides. Add enough liquid (broth, wine) to barely cover the brisket. Cook, covered, in a preheated 325°F (163°C) oven for 2½ to 3 hours. Slice thinly against the grain.

Tip: It is hard to beat brisket for flavor and texture. The leaner portion of brisket is called the flat, but the fattier section is tastiest.

Nutrition Facts		Amount Per 3-Ounce (85-Gram) Serving, (cooked)			
Calories	190	Total Carbohydrate*	0g 0%	Vitamin A*	0%
Calories from Fat 80		Dietary Fiber*	0g 0%	Vitamin C*	0%
Total Fat*	9g 15%	Sugars	0g	Calcium*	0%
Saturated Fat*	3g 15%	Protein	25g	Iron*	15%
Cholesterol*	80mg 25%	Potassium	242mg	* Percent Daily Values are based on a 2,000 calorie diet. Your daily values may be higher or lower, depending on your calorie needs.	
Sodium*	60mg 2%				

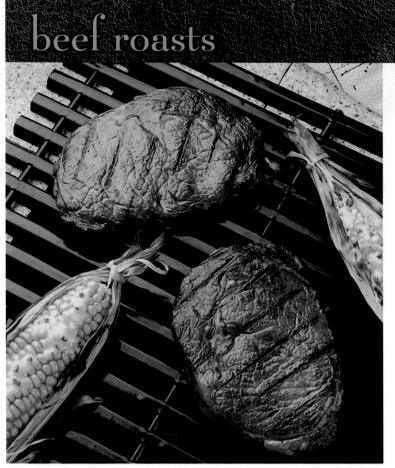

Rib Eye Steaks

Rib Steak, Small End
(Rib Grilling Steak, Small End)

- Pan-broil a 1-inch-thick (2.54cm) steak 11 to 14 minutes for medium rare. Turn once.
- Broil a 1-inch-thick (2.54cm) steak 13 to 17 minutes for medium rare. Turn once.
- Grill a 1-inch-thick (2.54cm) steak 9 to 12 minutes for medium rare. Turn once.

Tip: Cut from the small end of a standing rib roast, steaks from the rib section are of excellent quality. Before pan broiling wipe steak dry and it will brown quickly and evenly.

Nutrition Facts		Amount Per 3-Ounce (85-Gram) Serving, (cooked)			
Calories	190	Total Carbohydrate* 0g	0%	Vitamin A*	0%
Calories from Fat 90		Dietary Fiber* 0g	0%	Vitamin C*	0%
Total Fat*	10g 15%	Sugars 0g		Calcium*	2%
Saturated Fat*	4g 20%	Protein 24g		Iron*	10%
Cholesterol*	70mg 23%	Potassium 335mg		* Percent Daily Values are based on a 2,000 calorie diet. Your daily values may be higher or lower, depending on your calorie needs.	
Sodium*	60mg 3%				

Top Loin Steak, Boneless
(Strip Loin Grilling Steak, Boneless)

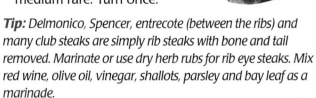

- Pan-broil a 1-inch-thick (2.54cm) steak 12 to 15 minutes for medium rare. Turn once.
- Broil a 1-inch-thick (2.54cm) steak 13 to 17 minutes for medium rare. Turn once.
- Grill a 1-inch-thick (2.54cm) steak 15 to 18 minutes for medium rare. Turn once.

Tip: Remove steak from the refrigerator at least an hour before cooking. To cook to desired doneness, use the "touch test": Rare is soft, medium has a slight give and well-done is firm.

Nutrition Facts		Amount Per 3-Ounce (85-Gram) Serving, (cooked)			
Calories	220	Total Carbohydrate* 0g	0%	Vitamin A*	0%
Calories from Fat 120		Dietary Fiber* 0g	0%	Vitamin C*	0%
Total Fat*	13g 20%	Sugars 0g		Calcium*	0%
Saturated Fat*	5g 25%	Protein 24g		Iron*	15%
Cholesterol*	75mg 25%	Potassium 310mg		* Percent Daily Values are based on a 2,000 calorie diet. Your daily values may be higher or lower, depending on your calorie needs.	
Sodium*	55mg 2%				

Rib Eye Steak, Boneless
(Rib Eye Grilling Steak, Boneless)

- Pan-broil a 1-inch-thick (2.54cm) steak 12 to 15 minutes for medium rare. Turn once.
- Broil a 1-inch-thick (2.54cm) steak 14 to 18 minutes for medium rare. Turn once.
- Grill a 1-inch-thick (2.54cm) steak 11 to 14 minutes for medium rare. Turn once.

Tip: Delmonico, Spencer, entrecote (between the ribs) and many club steaks are simply rib steaks with bone and tail removed. Marinate or use dry herb rubs for rib eye steaks. Mix red wine, olive oil, vinegar, shallots, parsley and bay leaf as a marinade.

Nutrition Facts		Amount Per 3-Ounce (85-Gram) Serving, (cooked)			
Calories	170	Total Carbohydrate* 0g	0%	Vitamin A*	0%
Calories from Fat 70		Dietary Fiber* 0g	0%	Vitamin C*	0%
Total Fat*	8g 12%	Sugars 0g		Calcium*	2%
Saturated Fat*	3g 15%	Protein 25g		Iron*	10%
Cholesterol*	75mg 25%	Potassium 310mg		* Percent Daily Values are based on a 2,000 calorie diet. Your daily values may be higher or lower, depending on your calorie needs.	
Sodium*	50mg 2%				

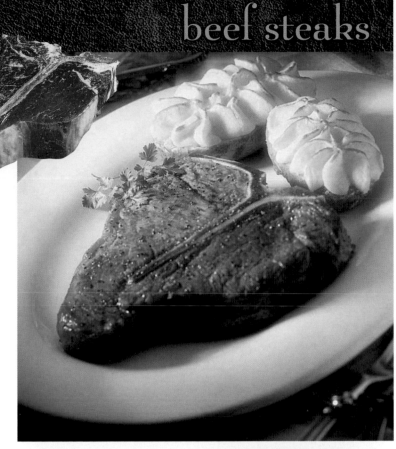

Porterhouse/T-Bone Steak
(Porterhouse/T-Bone Grilling Steak)

- Pan-broil a 1-inch-thick (2.54cm) steak 14 to 17 minutes for medium rare. Turn once.
- Broil a 1-inch-thick (2.54cm) steak 15 to 20 minutes for medium rare. Turn once.
- Grill a 1-inch-thick (2.54cm) steak 14 to 16 minutes for medium rare. Turn once.

Tip: Porterhouse steak was named for a New York porter and ale house in the early 1800s. Both are bone-in steaks from the tenderloin, but the porterhouse has more tenderloin area.

Nutrition Facts		Amount Per 3-Ounce (85-Gram) Serving, (cooked)			
Calories	150	Total Carbohydrate* 0g	0%	Vitamin A*	0%
Calories from Fat 60		Dietary Fiber* 0g	0%	Vitamin C*	0%
Total Fat*	6g 10%	Sugars 0g		Calcium*	0%
Saturated Fat*	2.5g 10%	Protein 22g		Iron*	15%
Cholesterol*	45mg 15%	Potassium 321mg		* Percent Daily Values are based on a 2,000 calorie diet. Your daily values may be higher or lower, depending on your calorie needs.	
Sodium*	60mg 2%				

Porterhouse/T-Bone Steak

Top Loin Steak, Bone-In
(Strip Loin Grilling Steak, Bone-In)

- Pan-broil a 1-inch-thick (2.54cm) steak 12 to 15 minutes for medium rare. Turn once.
- Broil a 1-inch-thick (2.54cm) steak 13 to 17 minutes for medium rare. Turn once.
- Grill a 1-inch-thick (2.54cm) steak 15 to 18 minutes for medium rare. Turn once.

Tip: This is the same as a New York strip. Aging beef accentuates the rich, beefy taste and increases tenderness. Dry-aged beef is rare and usually limited to rib and loin cuts.

Nutrition Facts		Amount Per 3-Ounce (85-Gram) Serving, (cooked)			
Calories	220	Total Carbohydrate* 0g	0%	Vitamin A*	0%
Calories from Fat 120		Dietary Fiber* 0g	0%	Vitamin C*	0%
Total Fat*	13g 20%	Sugars 0g		Calcium*	0%
Saturated Fat*	5g 25%	Protein 24g		Iron*	15%
Cholesterol*	75mg 25%	Potassium 310mg		* Percent Daily Values are based on a 2,000 calorie diet. Your daily values may be higher or lower, depending on your calorie needs.	
Sodium*	55mg 2%				

Filet Mignon
(Beef Tenderloin)

- Pan-broil 1-inch-thick (2.54cm) steaks in a heavy skillet brushed with oil to prevent sticking. Cook 10 to 13 minutes for medium rare. Turn once.
- Broil 1½-inch-thick (3.81cm) steaks 18 to 22 minutes for medium rare. Turn once.
- Grill 1½-inch-thick (3.81cm) steaks 14 to 16 minutes for medium rare. Turn once.

Tip: When wrapping bacon around fillets, overlap and secure the ends with a toothpick. A whole fillet or tenderloin weighs about 6 pounds (2.73kg) and serves 10 to 12 people.

Nutrition Facts		Amount Per 3-Ounce (85-Gram) Serving, (cooked)			
Calories	230	Total Carbohydrate* 0g	0%	Vitamin A*	0%
Calories from Fat 140		Dietary Fiber* 0g	0%	Vitamin C*	0%
Total Fat*	15g 23%	Sugars 0g		Calcium*	2%
Saturated Fat*	6g 30%	Protein 22g		Iron*	8%
Cholesterol*	80mg 27%	Potassium 270mg		* Percent Daily Values are based on a 2,000 calorie diet. Your daily values may be higher or lower, depending on your calorie needs.	
Sodium*	45mg 2%				

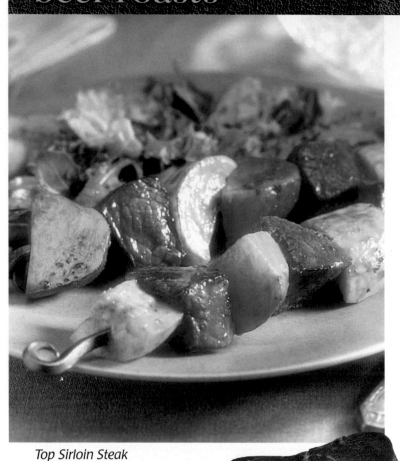

Top Sirloin Steak

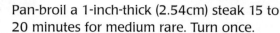

Tri Tip Steak
(Bottom Sirloin Grilling Steak)

- Pan-broil a 1-inch-thick (2.54cm) steak 15 to 20 minutes for medium rare. Turn once.
- Broil a 2-pound (.91kg) steak 16 to 21 minutes for medium rare. Turn once.
- Grill a 2-pound (.91kg) steak 17 to 21 minutes for medium rare. Turn once.

Tip: This is from a triangular cut from the bottom sirloin area. To pan-broil, preheat the skillet. Pour off fat as it accumulates or the steak will be fried. Serve steak as soon as juice appears on cooked side.

Nutrition Facts		Amount Per 3-Ounce (85-Gram) Serving, (cooked)			
Calories	210	Total Carbohydrate* 0g	0%	Vitamin A*	0%
Calories from Fat 100		Dietary Fiber* 0g	0%	Vitamin C*	0%
Total Fat*	11g 17%	Sugars 0g		Calcium*	2%
Saturated Fat*	4g 20%	Protein 26g		Iron*	20%
Cholesterol*	55mg 18%	Potassium 385mg		* Percent Daily Values are based on a 2,000 calorie diet. Your daily values may be higher or lower, depending on your calorie needs.	
Sodium*	60mg 3%				

Sirloin Steak, Boneless
(Sirloin Grilling Steak, Boneless)

- Pan-broil a 1-inch-thick (2.54cm) steak 15 to 20 minutes for medium rare. Turn once.
- Broil a 1-inch-thick (2.54cm) steak 16 to 21 minutes for medium rare. Turn once.
- Grill a 1-inch-thick (2.54cm) steak 17 to 21 minutes for medium rare. Turn once.

Tip: Use tongs for turning steaks on a grill; if pierced with a fork, they lose juiciness. A British king was credited with honoring his favorite meat by dubbing the steak "Sir Loin."

Nutrition Facts		Amount Per 3-Ounce (85-Gram) Serving, (cooked)			
Calories	220	Total Carbohydrate* 0g	0%	Vitamin A*	0%
Calories from Fat 120		Dietary Fiber* 0g	0%	Vitamin C*	0%
Total Fat*	13g 20%	Sugars 0g		Calcium*	2%
Saturated Fat*	5g 25%	Protein 23g		Iron*	8%
Cholesterol*	70mg 23%	Potassium 280mg		* Percent Daily Values are based on a 2,000 calorie diet. Your daily values may be higher or lower, depending on your calorie needs.	
Sodium*	45mg 2%				

Top Sirloin Steak, Boneless
(Top Loin Grilling Steak, Boneless)

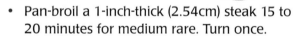

- Pan-broil a 1-inch-thick (2.54cm) steak 15 to 20 minutes for medium rare. Turn once.
- Broil a 1-inch-thick (2.54cm) steak 16 to 21 minutes for medium rare. Turn once.
- Grill a 1-inch-thick (2.54cm) steak for 17 to 21 minutes for medium rare. Turn once.

Tip: The sirloin is a cut from the hip area, lean and can be dry. Add a wet or dry marinade. Try mesquite or hickory wood chips when grilling for more flavor. Mesquite's sweet taste perfectly accents beef, while hickory adds a southern accent.

Nutrition Facts		Amount Per 3-Ounce (85-Gram) Serving, (cooked)			
Calories	150	Total Carbohydrate* 0g	0%	Vitamin A*	0%
Calories from Fat 45		Dietary Fiber* 0g	0%	Vitamin C*	0%
Total Fat*	4.5g 8%	Sugars 0g		Calcium*	0%
Saturated Fat*	2g 10%	Protein 26g		Iron*	15%
Cholesterol*	75mg 25%	Potassium 343mg		* Percent Daily Values are based on a 2,000 calorie diet. Your daily values may be higher or lower, depending on your calorie needs.	
Sodium*	55mg 2%				

Round Steak, Boneless
(Round Marinating Steak, Boneless)

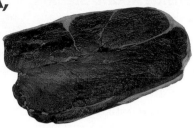

For Marinating:

- Ideal for braising, add ½ to 2 cups (118 to 473ml) liquid—wine or broth—with herbs to 1-inch-thick (2.54cm) browned steak. Cover tightly and cook in preheated 325°F (163°C) oven 1¾ to 2½ hours.

Tip: Generously add bay leaves, fresh thyme or rosemary, garlic, onions and mushrooms to braising liquid or marinades for round steak.

For Swissing:

- Dredge a 1-inch-thick (2.54cm) steak in seasoned flour. In a heavy, lidded casserole, brown the steak on both sides. Add ½ to 2 cups (118 to 473ml) liquid. Cover tightly and cook in preheated 325°F (163°C) oven 1¾ to 2½ hours.

Tip: Add sliced onions, sour cream, paprika and salt and pepper to the steak and liquid mixture.

Tip: Round steaks are very lean but not as tender and juicy as other cuts. Cut from the rear of the animal, they are less tender due to the relatively small amount of fat on the heavily exercised back muscles. Round steaks usually require a moist-heat cooking method. Because of this, they are often broiled, braised or cooked in a liquid. Top Round Steak (Inside Round Steak) on page 14 is a good substitute for Boneless Round Steak, but is usually a bit thicker).

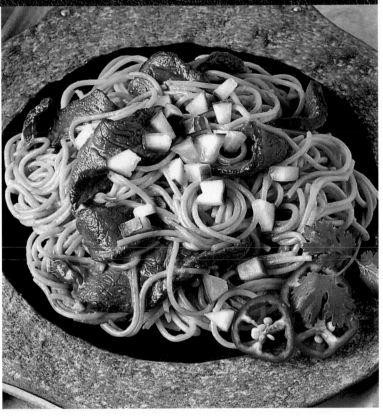

Round Steak

Top Blade Steak
(Top Blade Simmering Steak)

- Pat dry before pan broiling.
- Marinate steak.
- Pan-broil a 1-inch-thick (2.54cm) steak 13 to 17 minutes for medium rare. Turn once.
- Grill a 1-inch-thick (2.54cm) steak 18 to 22 minutes for medium rare. Turn once.

Tip: Also known as flatiron steaks, or blade steaks, the biggest disadvantage to this cut is a line of gristle down the center. Easily affordable, they are best marinated and grilled. The area where it comes from is shaped like an old-fashioned iron.

Nutrition Facts Amount Per 3-Ounce (85-Gram) Serving, (cooked)					
Calories	210	Total Carbohydrate* 0g	0%	Vitamin A*	0%
Calories from Fat 90		Dietary Fiber* 0g	0%	Vitamin C*	0%
Total Fat*	10g 15%	Sugars 0g		Calcium*	0%
Saturated Fat*	3.5g 18%	Protein 29g		Iron*	15%
Cholesterol*	75mg 25%	Potassium 270mg		* Percent Daily Values are based on a 2,000 calorie diet. Your daily values may be higher or lower, depending on your calorie needs.	
Sodium*	40mg 2%				

Nutrition Facts Amount Per 3-Ounce (85-Gram) Serving, (cooked)					
Calories	180	Total Carbohydrate* 0g	0%	Vitamin A*	0%
Calories from Fat 90		Dietary Fiber* 0g	0%	Vitamin C*	0%
Total Fat*	10g 15%	Sugars 0g		Calcium*	0%
Saturated Fat*	3g 15%	Protein 22g		Iron*	15%
Cholesterol*	50mg 17%	Potassium 260mg		* Percent Daily Values are based on a 2,000 calorie diet. Your daily values may be higher or lower, depending on your calorie needs.	
Sodium*	60mg 3%				

Flank Steak

Top Round Steak
(Inside Round Steak)

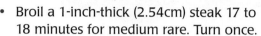

- Marinate to tenderize.
- Pan-broil a 1-inch-thick (2.54cm) steak 15 to 16 minutes for medium rare. Turn once.
- Broil a 1-inch-thick (2.54cm) steak 17 to 18 minutes for medium rare. Turn once.
- Grill a 1-inch-thick (2.54cm) steak for 16 to 18 minutes for medium rare. Turn once.

Tip: A light brushing of olive oil before grilling or broiling adds flavor and juiciness.

Nutrition Facts		Amount Per 3-Ounce (85-Gram) Serving, (cooked)			
Calories	180	Total Carbohydrate* 0g 0%		Vitamin A*	0%
Calories from Fat 80		Dietary Fiber* 0g 0%		Vitamin C*	0%
Total Fat*	8g 10%	Sugars	0g	Calcium*	0%
Saturated Fat*	3g 15%	Protein	26g	Iron*	15%
Cholesterol*	70mg 25%	Potassium	360mg	* Percent Daily Values are based on a 2,000 calorie diet. Your daily values may be higher or lower, depending on your calorie needs.	
Sodium*	50mg 2%				

Eye of Round Steak
(Rib Grilling Steak)

- In a heavy, lidded casserole, brown 4 1-inch-thick (2.54cm) steaks on all sides. Add ½ to 2 cups (118 to 473ml) of beef broth. Cover and simmer for 1¾ to 2½ hours or until tender.

Tip: Always braise round steaks for tenderness. They do not respond to dry heat methods.

Flank Steak
(Flank Marinating Steak)

- Marinate to tenderize.
- Broil 13 to 18 minutes for medium rare depending on thickness. Turn once.
- Grill 17 to 21 minutes for medium rare depending on thickness. Turn once.

Tip: The acidic ingredients in many marinades, such as vinegar and soy sauce, help to tenderize flank steak. Another delicious alternative marinade is teriyaki. Use a kitchen fork to prick holes in both sides of flank steak. Refrigerate flank steak in teriyaki at least six hours or overnight. Turn halfway through marinating time.

Nutrition Facts		Amount Per 3-Ounce (85-Gram) Serving, (cooked)			
Calories	150	Total Carbohydrate* 0g 0%		Vitamin A*	0%
Calories from Fat 40		Dietary Fiber* 0g 0%		Vitamin C*	0%
Total Fat*	4.5g 7%	Sugars	0g	Calcium*	0%
Saturated Fat*	1.5g 8%	Protein	25g	Iron*	10%
Cholesterol*	60mg 20%	Potassium	205mg	* Percent Daily Values are based on a 2,000 calorie diet. Your daily values may be higher or lower, depending on your calorie needs.	
Sodium*	35mg 1%				

Nutrition Facts		Amount Per 3-Ounce (85-Gram) Serving, (cooked)			
Calories	180	Total Carbohydrate* 0g 0%		Vitamin A*	0%
Calories from Fat 80		Dietary Fiber* 0g 0%		Vitamin C*	0%
Total Fat*	9g 15%	Sugars	0g	Calcium*	0%
Saturated Fat*	3.5g 20%	Protein	23g	Iron*	10%
Cholesterol*	55mg 20%	Potassium	352mg	* Percent Daily Values are based on a 2,000 calorie diet. Your daily values may be higher or lower, depending on your calorie needs.	
Sodium*	70mg 2%				

Skirt Steak
(Skirt Marinating Steak)

- Pat steaks dry.
- Marinate a 1½-pound (.68kg) steak.
- Pan-broil 7 to 9 minutes for medium rare. Turn once.
- Broil 8 to 10 minutes for medium rare. Turn once.
- Grill 7 to 9 minutes for medium rare. Turn once.

Tip: Skirt steak is actually the diaphragm of beef. It has coarse texture and a rich, beefy taste. Marinate to allow loose grain to absorb flavor. It is the authentic meat for fajitas.

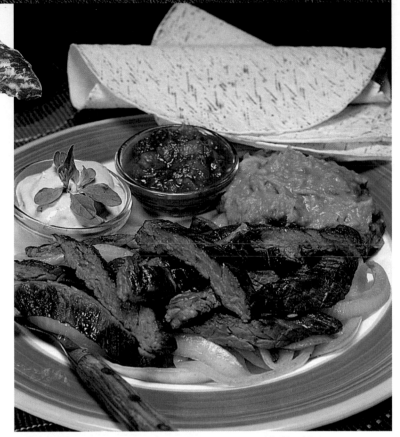

Skirt Steak

Nutrition Facts Amount Per 3-Ounce (85-Gram) Serving, (cooked)

Calories	170	Total Carbohydrate* 0g	0%	Vitamin A*	0%
Calories from Fat 80		Dietary Fiber* 0g	0%	Vitamin C*	0%
Total Fat*	9g 14%	Sugars 0g		Calcium*	0%
Saturated Fat*	3.5g 18%	Protein 23g		Iron*	15%
Cholesterol*	50mg 17%	Potassium 250mg			
Sodium*	65mg 3%				

* Percent Daily Values are based on a 2,000 calorie diet. Your daily values may be higher or lower, depending on your calorie needs.

Back Ribs
(Grilling Back Ribs)

- Preheat oven to 350°F (177°C). Liberally sprinkle 4 to 5 pounds (1.82 to 2.27kg) of ribs with garlic powder, salt and pepper. Roast 45 minutes to 1 hour.

Tip: The meat on beef ribs is tender and flavorful. Try a dry rub; grill over coals 10 minutes per side, adding barbecue sauce just at the end. Combine thyme, rosemary, paprika, salt and pepper as a dry rub.

Short Ribs, English Cut
(Simmering Short Ribs, English Cut)

- Dredge ribs in seasoned flour. Brown short ribs on all sides. Add 2 cups (473ml) of beef broth or red wine. Cover and simmer for 1 hour or until fork-tender.

Tip: About 4 inches (10.16cm) of a rib roast is usually trimmed off, creating short ribs. Marinate to tenderize.

Nutrition Facts Amount Per 3-Ounce (85-Gram) Serving, (cooked)

Calories	300	Total Carbohydrate* 0g	0%	Vitamin A*	0%
Calories from Fat 220		Dietary Fiber* 0g	0%	Vitamin C*	0%
Total Fat*	24g 37%	Sugars 0g		Calcium*	0%
Saturated Fat*	10g 50%	Protein 19g		Iron*	10%
Cholesterol*	70mg 23%	Potassium 260mg			
Sodium*	55mg 2%				

* Percent Daily Values are based on a 2,000 calorie diet. Your daily values may be higher or lower, depending on your calorie needs.

Nutrition Facts Amount Per 3-Ounce (85-Gram) Serving, (cooked)

Calories	250	Total Carbohydrate* 0g	0%	Vitamin A*	0%
Calories from Fat 140		Dietary Fiber* 0g	0%	Vitamin C*	0%
Total Fat*	15g 25%	Sugars 0g		Calcium*	0%
Saturated Fat*	7g 35%	Protein 26g		Iron*	15%
Cholesterol*	80mg 25%	Potassium 266mg			
Sodium*	50mg 2%				

* Percent Daily Values are based on a 2,000 calorie diet. Your daily values may be higher or lower, depending on your calorie needs.

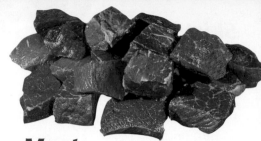

Beef Stew Meat
(Stewing Cubes)

- Dredge 3 pounds (1.36kg) of beef cubes in seasoned flour. Brown on all sides. Cover and simmer in 12 oz. (355ml or .75 pint) dark beer. Add onion, carrots, garlic, bay leaf and thyme. Simmer for 1½ hours or until fork-tender.

Tip: Alternatively, use beef broth or red wine for liquid. Other vegetable possibilities include using potatoes, parsnips, turnips or tomatoes.

Nutrition Facts	Amount Per 3-Ounce (85-Gram) Serving, (cooked)				
Calories	200	Total Carbohydrate*	0g 0%	Vitamin A*	0%
Calories from Fat 90		Dietary Fiber*	0g 0%	Vitamin C*	0%
Total Fat*	10g 15%	Sugars	0g	Calcium*	0%
Saturated Fat*	4g 18%	Protein	27g	Iron*	15%
Cholesterol*	85mg 28%	Potassium	235mg	* Percent Daily Values are based on a 2,000 calorie diet. Your daily values may be higher or lower, depending on your calorie needs.	
Sodium*	55mg 2%				

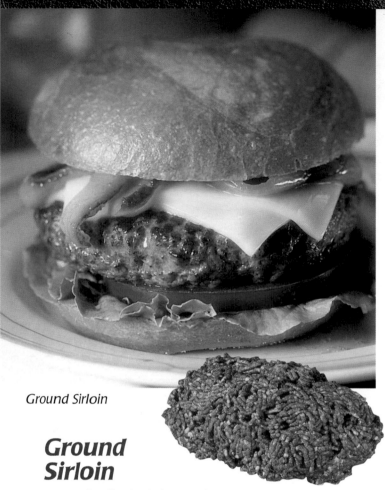

Ground Sirloin

Ground Sirloin

- Pan-broil ¾-inch (1.91cm) patties over medium-high heat for 10 minutes or until the internal temperature reaches 160°F (71°C). Turn once.

- Broil ¾-inch (1.91cm) patties 3 inches (7.62cm) from the heat source for 10 minutes or until the internal temperature reaches 160°F (71°C). Turn once.

- Grill ¾-inch (1.91cm) patties over medium-hot coals for 10 minutes or until the internal temperature reaches 160°F (71°C). Turn once.

Tip: To 2 pounds (.91kg) ground sirloin, add one package of dry onion soup mix. Other options include adding garlic, Worcestershire or Dijon mustard to flavor patties before cooking.

Nutrition Facts	Amount Per 3-Ounce (85-Gram) Serving, (cooked)				
Calories	230	Total Carbohydrate*	0g 0%	Vitamin A*	0%
Calories from Fat 140		Dietary Fiber*	0g 0%	Vitamin C*	0%
Total Fat*	16g 25%	Sugars	0g	Calcium*	0%
Saturated Fat*	6g 30%	Protein	21g	Iron*	10%
Cholesterol*	75mg 25%	Potassium	256mg	* Percent Daily Values are based on a 2,000 calorie diet. Your daily values may be higher or lower, depending on your calorie needs.	
Sodium*	65mg 2%				

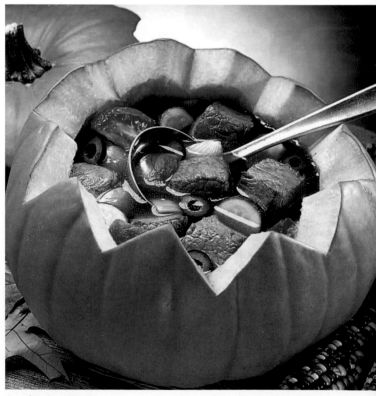

Beef Stew Meat

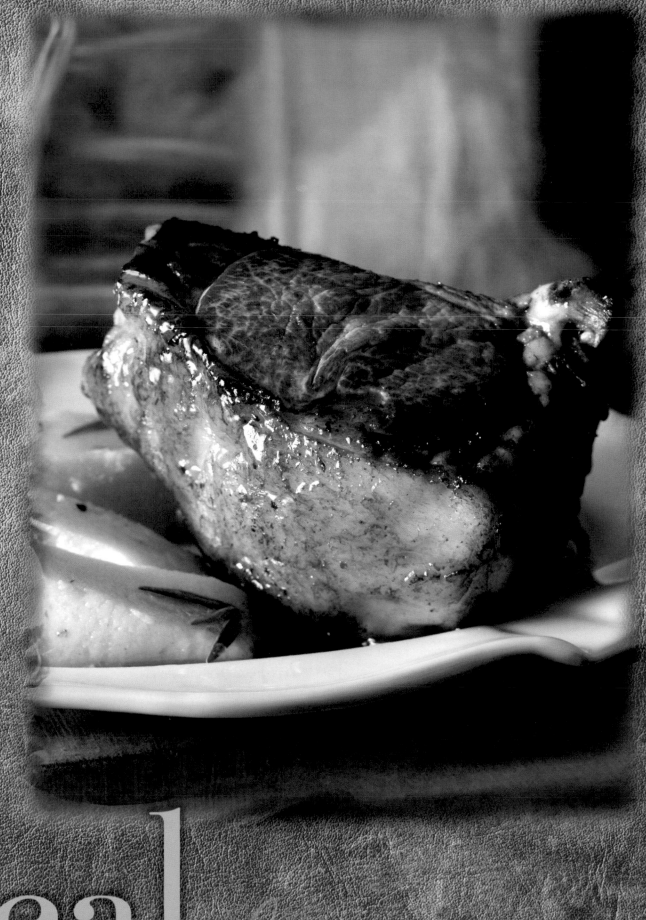

veal

What is veal?

Veal is meat from calves up to 6 months old. It is very delicate, lean meat. Veal has less fat than boneless, skinless chicken breast.

What is formula-fed (milk-fed and special-fed) veal?

This veal comes from an animal between 18 and 20 weeks old, weighing up to 525 pounds (239kg). It has been raised on a formula of skim milk, protein, vitamins and minerals.

What is veal scallopini?

This is the Italian term for thin slices of veal that can be cooked quickly. Veal scallopini should be ¼ to ⅜ of an inch (.64 to .96cm) thick. If cut more thinly, it will dry out in the time it takes to cook.

Should veal be marinated?

Yes, sometimes. The flavor of veal is mild. When grilled, dry rubs and marinades enhance its flavor. Marinate only in the refrigerator, never on the counter to prevent foodborne illness.

What are sweetbreads?

These are veal glands, such as the thymus or the pancreas. They are considered a delicacy.

What is the difference between calf's liver and beef liver?

Calf's liver is more delicate and milder than beef liver.

SELECTION

- Choose veal that is creamy pink in color and that has a fine-grained texture.
- Bones should be white with a bright red center.
- Look for fat that is milky white, not yellow.
- Veal should be moist, but not wet. The meat should be firm with no marbling.

STORAGE

- When shopping, select your meat last to ensure that the veal stays as cold as possible.
- If it will not be refrigerated within 30 minutes, place the veal in a cooler.
- Keep veal in the coldest part of your refrigerator.
- If you don't plan to use the veal within 2 days, freeze it immediately.
- Ground meats are more perishable than roasts or steaks. Use them within 1 day.
- When freezing multiple packages, spread them out. Do not stack on top of each other.
- Prevent freezer burn by re-wrapping the meat in moisture-proof, airtight material, such as food freezer bags or heavy-duty aluminum foil.

HANDLING

- Wash hands with hot soapy water for 20 seconds before and after handling veal.
- Wash knives, counters and cutting boards in hot soapy water immediately after any meat contact.
- Do not use the meat knife to cut vegetables without washing the knife and cutting board first. Wiping is not sufficient to kill bacteria.
- Never place cooked veal back on the same platter that held raw meat.
- Always defrost veal in the refrigerator.
- Pat veal steaks, cubes and roasts dry with a paper towel for better browning.

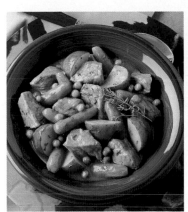

Veal Stew Meat

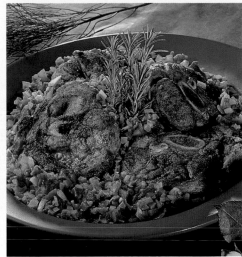

Veal Shanks

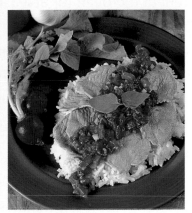

Veal Scallopini

VEAL CUT	PAN-BROIL	ROAST	GRILL	PAN-FRY SAUTÉ	BRAISE
Calf's Liver				X	
Loin Chops	X		X		
Rib Chops	X		X		
Veal Blade Roast		X			X
Veal, Ground	X	Meat Loaf	X	X	
Veal Leg Roast, Boneless		X			
Veal Loin Roast, Boneless		X			
Veal Rib Roast		X			
Veal Scallopini/Cutlets				X	
Veal Sirloin Roast		X			
Veal Shanks					X
Veal Stew Meat					X

(Broiling veal is not recommended.)

How to roast

- Preheat the oven for at least 10 minutes.
- Cook roasts fat side up.
- Use an instant-read thermometer. Insert halfway into roast, making sure not to touch bone.
- Remove roast from oven when the internal temperature reaches 155°F (68°C).
- Always allow roast to rest 10 to 15 minutes after cooking before slicing. The temperature will increase a few degrees. Cover loosely with a tent of aluminum foil.

How to grill chops

- Use medium ash-covered coals to grill.
- Let chops rest a few minutes for optimum juiciness.

Recommended marinades and dry rubs for veal chops

MARINADES:

- Olive oil, crushed garlic, salt and pepper
- Olive oil, balsamic vinegar and crushed garlic
- White wine, minced shallots, oil and fresh tarragon
- Mustard, white wine, thyme and ginger

DRY RUBS (rub the chops with olive oil first so the seasonings will stick):

- Cumin, chili powder, black pepper and brown sugar
- Paprika, chili powder, garlic powder, mustard and brown sugar
- Thyme, sage, salt and pepper

How to sauté and pan-broil

- To sauté/pan-fry, cook over medium-high heat in 2 tablespoons (30ml) of oil for a short time. Do not add water; do not cover.
- To pan-broil, cook over medium heat in a heavy nonstick skillet. Do not add oil or water; do not cover.

How to braise

- To braise, sear veal on all sides in a heavy, lidded casserole. Add ½ to 2 cups (118 to 473ml) of liquid. Bring to a boil; reduce heat. Cover tightly and simmer gently over low heat on top of range or in a preheated 325°F (163°C) oven until veal is fork-tender.

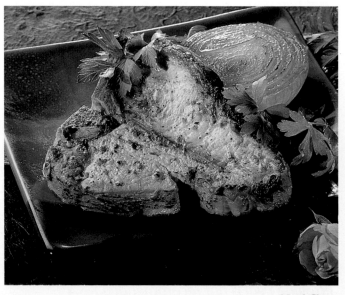

Veal Chop

Veal Blade Roast

- Brown roast and desired vegetables in a heavy, lidded casserole. Add ½ to 2 cups (118 to 473ml) of liquid. Cover and cook in a preheated 325°F (163°C) oven until meat is fork-tender.

- Roast on rack in roasting pan in a preheated 325°F (163°C) oven to internal temperature of 145°F (63°C) for an ideal medium doneness. Veal should be moist and faintly pink in the center. Let roast rest 15 to 20 minutes before carving.

Tip: Rubs are a savory way to bring out the flavor of veal roasts; experiment with different herb combinations.

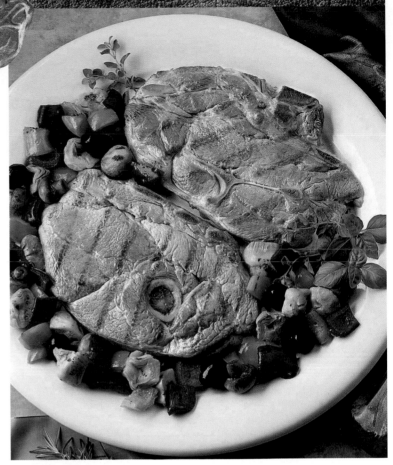

Veal Blade Roast

Nutrition Facts	Amount Per 3-Ounce (85-Gram) Serving, (cooked)				
Calories	150	Total Carbohydrate* 0g	0%	Vitamin A*	0%
Calories from Fat 50		Dietary Fiber* 0g	0%	Vitamin C*	0%
Total Fat*	6g 8%	Sugars 0g		Calcium*	2%
Saturated Fat*	2g 10%	Protein 22g		Iron*	4%
Cholesterol* 100mg	35%	Potassium 264mg		* Percent Daily Values are based on a 2,000 calorie diet. Your daily values may be higher or lower, depending on your calorie needs.	
Sodium* 85mg	4%				

Veal Loin Roast, Boneless

- Roast in a preheated 325°F (163°C) oven to an internal temperature of 145°F (63°C). Let roast rest 15 to 20 minutes before carving.

Tip: Rub with paste of olive oil, shallots, fresh sage and salt and pepper.

Veal Rib Roast

- Roast a rib roast in a preheated 325°F (163°C) oven to an internal temperature of 145°F (63°C). Let roast rest 15 to 20 minutes before carving.

Tip: Veal has very little waste. Select delicate, creamy pink veal with milk-white fat. Veal rib, rack, leg and loin roasts are excellent roasted.

Nutrition Facts	Amount Per 3-Ounce (85-Gram) Serving, (cooked)				
Calories	150	Total Carbohydrate* 0g	0%	Vitamin A*	0%
Calories from Fat 60		Dietary Fiber* 0g	0%	Vitamin C*	0%
Total Fat*	6g 10%	Sugars 0g		Calcium*	0%
Saturated Fat*	2g 10%	Protein 22g		Iron*	4%
Cholesterol* 90mg	30%	Potassium 289mg		* Percent Daily Values are based on a 2,000 calorie diet. Your daily values may be higher or lower, depending on your calorie needs.	
Sodium* 80mg	4%				

Nutrition Facts	Amount Per 3-Ounce (85-Gram) Serving, (cooked)				
Calories	150	Total Carbohydrate* 0g	0%	Vitamin A*	0%
Calories from Fat 60		Dietary Fiber* 0g	0%	Vitamin C*	0%
Total Fat*	6g 10%	Sugars 0g		Calcium*	0%
Saturated Fat*	2g 8%	Protein 22g		Iron*	4%
Cholesterol* 100mg	35%	Potassium 264mg		* Percent Daily Values are based on a 2,000 calorie diet. Your daily values may be higher or lower, depending on your calorie needs.	
Sodium* 80mg	4%				

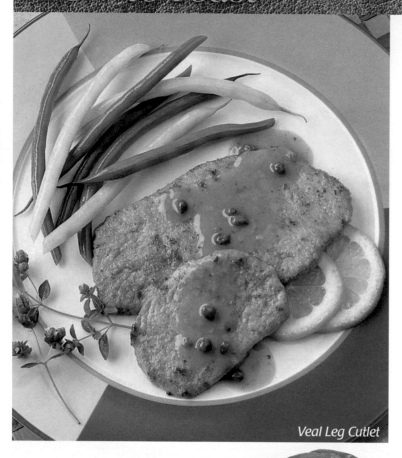

Veal Leg Cutlet

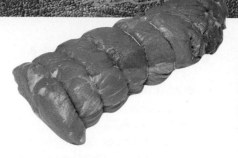

Veal Leg Roast, Boneless

- Roast in a preheated 325°F (163°C) oven for 25 to 30 minutes per pound (.45kg) to an internal temperature of 145°F (63°C) for medium doneness. Let roast rest 15 to 20 minutes.

Tip: Delicious, but slightly expensive, another option for leg roast is braising in liquid laced with leeks, carrots, fresh thyme and bacon.

Nutrition Facts	Amount Per 3-Ounce (85-Gram) Serving, (cooked)			
Calories	130	Total Carbohydrate* 0g 0%	Vitamin A*	0%
Calories from Fat 25		Dietary Fiber* 0g 0%	Vitamin C*	0%
Total Fat*	3g 4%	Sugars 0g	Calcium*	0%
Saturated Fat*	1g 6%	Protein 24g	Iron*	4%
Cholesterol*	90mg 30%	Potassium 334mg	* Percent Daily Values are based on a 2,000 calorie diet. Your daily values may be higher or lower, depending on your calorie needs.	
Sodium*	60mg 2%			

Veal Sirloin Roast

- Roast in a preheated 325°F (163°C) oven for 45 minutes to 1 hour to an internal temperature of 145°F (63°C). Let roast rest 15 to 20 minutes before carving.

Tip: Choose veal that is creamy pink in color with fine-grained texture and milky white fat, firm with no marbling.

Nutrition Facts	Amount Per 3-Ounce (85-Gram) Serving, (cooked)			
Calories	140	Total Carbohydrate* 0g 0%	Vitamin A*	0%
Calories from Fat 50		Dietary Fiber* 0g 0%	Vitamin C*	0%
Total Fat*	5g 8%	Sugars 0g	Calcium*	0%
Saturated Fat*	2g 10%	Protein 22g	Iron*	4%
Cholesterol*	90mg 30%	Potassium 310mg	* Percent Daily Values are based on a 2,000 calorie diet. Your daily values may be higher or lower, depending on your calorie needs.	
Sodium*	70mg 4%			

Veal Rib Roast

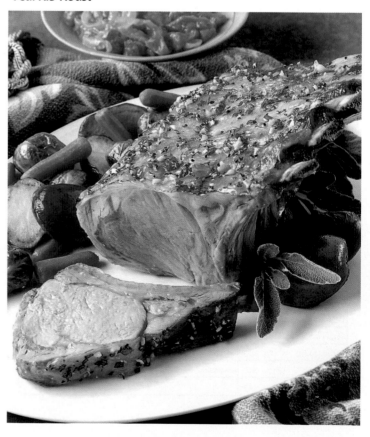

Loin Chops

- Grill 1-inch-thick (2.54cm) chops over medium-hot coals for 12 to 14 minutes for medium rare. Add 2 to 4 minutes for medium. Turn once.
- Sauté 1-inch-thick (2.54cm) chops. Cook over medium-high heat for 10 to 14 minutes for medium rare. Turn once.

Tip: Before cooking, try brushing both sides of chops with olive oil to seal in veal's delicate flavor and juices.

Nutrition Facts		Amount Per 3-Ounce (85-Gram) Serving, (cooked)			
Calories	160	Total Carbohydrate*	0g 0%	Vitamin A*	0%
Calories from Fat	60	Dietary Fiber*	0g 0%	Vitamin C*	0%
Total Fat*	7g 10%	Sugars	0g	Calcium*	0%
Saturated Fat*	2.5g 15%	Protein	23g	Iron*	10%
Cholesterol*	70mg 25%	Potassium	301mg	* Percent Daily Values are based on a 2,000 calorie diet. Your daily values may be higher or lower, depending on your calorie needs.	
Sodium*	55mg 2%				

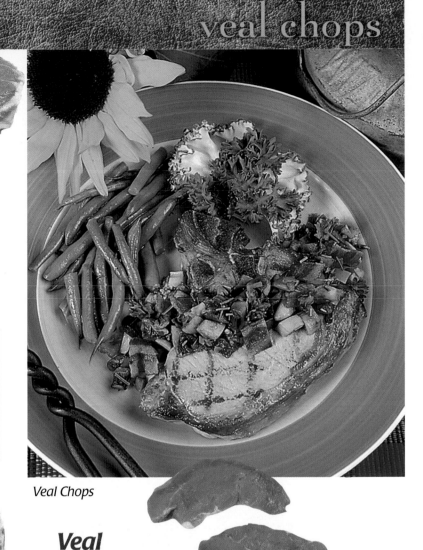

Veal Chops

Rib Chops

- Grill 1-inch-thick (2.54cm) rib chops over medium hot coals for 12 to 14 minutes for medium rare. Add 3 to 4 minutes for medium. Turn once.
- Sauté 1-inch-thick (2.54cm) rib chops in 2 tablespoons (30ml) of oil over medium-high heat for 10 to 14 minutes. Turn once.

Tip: Firm meat with adequate fat, rib chops are sold with bone and rib piece or boneless.

Nutrition Facts		Amount Per 3-Ounce (85-Gram) Serving, (cooked)			
Calories	210	Total Carbohydrate*	0g 0%	Vitamin A*	0%
Calories from Fat	100	Dietary Fiber*	0g 0%	Vitamin C*	0%
Total Fat*	11g 17%	Sugars	0g	Calcium*	2%
Saturated Fat*	4g 20%	Protein	28g	Iron*	6%
Cholesterol*	120mg 40%	Potassium	260mg	* Percent Daily Values are based on a 2,000 calorie diet. Your daily values may be higher or lower, depending on your calorie needs.	
Sodium*	80mg 3%				

Veal Scallopini (Cutlets)

- Dredge ¼-inch-thick (.64cm) scallopini in flour. Shake off excess. Heat 1½ tablespoons (22ml) of oil in a pan over high heat. Add the veal (cook in batches). Cook 2 to 3 minutes until small beads of liquid appear on top of the veal. Turn and cook 2 to 3 more minutes.

Tip: Panko, or Japanese bread crumbs, makes an excellent breading for veal cutlets; look for it in Asian grocery stores.

Nutrition Facts		Amount Per 3-Ounce (85-Gram) Serving, (cooked)			
Calories	170	Total Carbohydrate*	0g 0%	Vitamin A*	0%
Calories from Fat	50	Dietary Fiber*	0g 0%	Vitamin C*	0%
Total Fat*	6g 8%	Sugars	0g	Calcium*	2%
Saturated Fat*	1.5g 8%	Protein	27g	Iron*	6%
Cholesterol*	100mg 35%	Potassium	287mg	* Percent Daily Values are based on a 2,000 calorie diet. Your daily values may be higher or lower, depending on your calorie needs.	
Sodium*	75mg 4%				

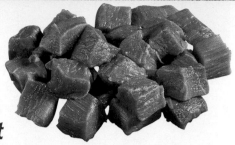

Veal Stew Meat

- Brown cubes and desired vegetables in a heavy, lidded casserole. Add ½ to 2 cups (118 to 473ml) of liquid. Simmer on the stove until tender.

Tip: Veal breast bones add extra body and flavor to stews.

Nutrition Facts	Amount Per 3-Ounce (85-Gram) Serving, (cooked)				
Calories	170	Total Carbohydrate*	0g	0%	Vitamin A*	0%
Calories from Fat	50	Dietary Fiber*	0g	0%	Vitamin C*	0%
Total Fat*	6g	8%	Sugars	0g	Calcium*	2%
Saturated Fat*	1.5g	8%	Protein	27g	Iron*	6%
Cholesterol*	100mg	35%	Potassium	287mg	* Percent Daily Values are based on a 2,000 calorie diet. Your daily values may be higher or lower, depending on your calorie needs.
Sodium*	75mg	4%			

Veal Shanks

- Brown meaty shanks in a heavy, lidded casserole. Add ½ to 2 cups (118 to 473ml) of liquid. Cover and cook in a preheated 325°F (163°C) oven for 1¼ to 2 hours or until tender.

Tip: Substitute veal shanks for lamb shanks in recipes. Use veal shanks to make flavored broth.

Nutrition Facts	Amount Per 3-Ounce (85-Gram) Serving, (cooked)				
Calories	150	Total Carbohydrate*	0g	0%	Vitamin A*	0%
Calories from Fat	35	Dietary Fiber*	0g	0%	Vitamin C*	0%
Total Fat*	3.5g	6%	Sugars	0g	Calcium*	2%
Saturated Fat*	1g	4%	Protein	27g	Iron*	6%
Cholesterol*	105mg	35%	Potassium	263mg	* Percent Daily Values are based on a 2,000 calorie diet. Your daily values may be higher or lower, depending on your calorie needs.
Sodium*	80mg	4%			

Ground Veal

- Sauté 4 veal patties (½ inch or 1.27cm thick) in 2 tablespoons (30ml) of oil over medium-high heat for 5 to 7 minutes for medium and 6 to 9 minutes for well done.
- Brown 1 pound (.45kg) of veal meatballs, then cook in a preheated 350°F (177°C) oven for 10 minutes.

Tip: To lower fat, substitute veal meatballs for beef in your next pasta dish.

Nutrition Facts	Amount Per 3-Ounce (85-Gram) Serving, (cooked)				
Calories	150	Total Carbohydrate*	0g	0%	Vitamin A*	0%
Calories from Fat	60	Dietary Fiber*	0g	0%	Vitamin C*	0%
Total Fat*	6g	10%	Sugars	0g	Calcium*	0%
Saturated Fat*	2.5g	15%	Protein	21g	Iron*	4%
Cholesterol*	90mg	30%	Potassium	286mg	* Percent Daily Values are based on a 2,000 calorie diet. Your daily values may be higher or lower, depending on your calorie needs.
Sodium*	70mg	2%			

Calf's Liver

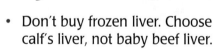

- Don't buy frozen liver. Choose calf's liver, not baby beef liver.
- Sauté 1½ pounds (.68kg) of calf's liver, thinly sliced, in 2 tablespoons (30ml) of oil over medium-high heat for 4 to 6 minutes, turning once.

Tip: Look for pale red to yellow-brown raw liver. Do not overcook organ meats. Liver should be slightly pink, delicate, tender and mild when cooked.

Nutrition Facts	Amount Per 3-Ounce (85-Gram) Serving, (cooked)				
Calories	140	Total Carbohydrate*	2g	0%	Vitamin A*	460%
Calories from Fat	50	Dietary Fiber*	0g	0%	Vitamin C*	45%
Total Fat*	6g	10%	Sugars	0g	Calcium*	0%
Saturated Fat*	2g	10%	Protein	18g	Iron*	10%
Cholesterol*	477mg	160%	Potassium	174mg	* Percent Daily Values are based on a 2,000 calorie diet. Your daily values may be higher or lower, depending on your calorie needs.
Sodium*	45mg	0%			

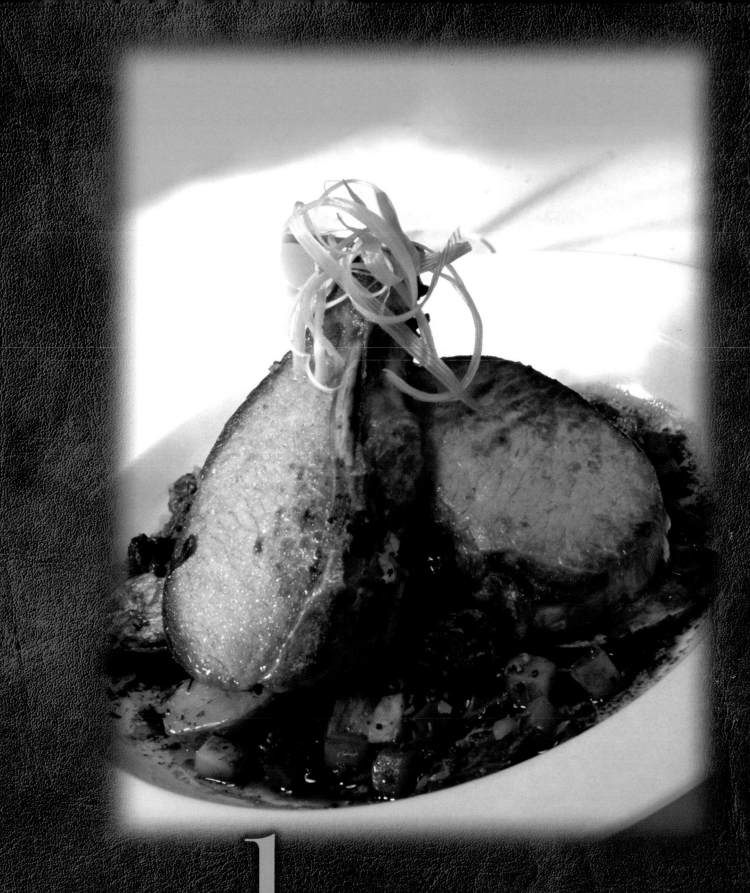

pork

When is pork done?

Chops and lean roasts should be taken off the heat at 145°F (63°C) and allowed to rest for 10 minutes. (The temperature will rise a few degrees while resting.) The United States Department of Agriculture recommends a serving temperature of 150°F (66°C) for ultimate safety.

Is ground pork done at 145°F to 150°F (63°C to 66°C)?

No. Ground pork should be cooked until the internal temperature reaches 155°F (68°C).

Why do older cookbooks recommend cooking pork to 180°F?

Today's pork is much leaner. Cooking pork to internal temperatures of 170°F to 180°F (77°C to 82°C) will result in dry, tough pork.

Is it safe to eat pork that is slightly pink in the middle?

Yes. The bacteria trichina is destroyed at 137°F (58°C). Pork cooked to a temperature of 145°F (63°C) will often have a slightly pink middle.

What's the difference between spareribs, back ribs and country-style ribs?

Spareribs have the least meat but are the most popular. Back ribs contain the rib bones and the "finger meat" between the ribs. Country-style ribs are very meaty.

When do you add the barbecue sauce to grilled meats?

The sugars in barbecue sauce will burn if they are put on the pork at the beginning of the grill time. Add the sauce during the last few minutes.

What is the leanest cut of pork?

The tenderloin is the leanest with only 4.1 grams of fat and 139 calories (580.32kJ) in a 3-ounce (85g) serving.

SELECTION

- Look for meat that is pale reddish pink. Any marbling should be creamy white, firm and smooth.
- Loin meat is paler than leg meat with the exception of the tenderloin which is a deep red. Pork loin should have a fine grain.
- Look for packages without any liquid. If there is liquid present, be sure it is clear, not cloudy. There should be no off odor.

STORAGE

- Purchase pork immediately before checkout. If the pork will not be refrigerated within 30 minutes, place it in a cooler.
- Store pork in the coldest part of the refrigerator. Pork can be refrigerated for 3 days and frozen for 4 to 6 months.
- The smaller the piece of pork, the faster it will spoil.
- If you don't plan to use the pork within a few days, freeze it immediately.
- Prevent freezer burn by re-wrapping the meat in moisture-proof, airtight material, such as food freezer bags or heavy-duty aluminum foil.

HANDLING

- Wash hands with hot soapy water for 20 seconds before and after handling pork.
- Do not use the meat knife to cut vegetables without washing the knife and cutting board first. Wiping is not sufficient to kill bacteria.
- Never place cooked pork back on the same platter used before cooking.
- Always defrost and marinate pork in the refrigerator, never on the counter.

PORK CUT	ROAST	GRILL	BROIL	PAN-BROIL	BRAISE
Blade Chop		X			X
Boston Butt Roast	X				X
Ham	X	X			X
Leg of Pork, Butt Half	X				
Leg of Pork, Shank End					X
Loin Chop		X	X	X	
Picnic Shoulder Arm Roast					X
Pork Chop		X	X	X	
Pork Chop, Smoked					X
Pork Crown Roast	X				
Pork Loin, Center-Cut, Boneless	X				
Pork Loin, Center-Cut, Bone-In	X				
Pork Tenderloin	X	X	X (Butterflied)	X	
Rib Chop		X	X	X	
Sirloin Chop, Boneless					X
Sirloin Pork Roast, Boneless	X				
Sirloin Pork Roast, Bone-In	X				
Whole Fresh Leg of Pork	X				

How to sauté and braise

- To sauté pork, cook in 2 tablespoons (30ml) of oil over medium-high heat for a short amount of time. Turn when juices are visible on the top side.

- To braise, brown pork on all sides to seal in juices. Brown desired vegetables. Place pork and vegetables in a heavy, lidded casserole. Add 2 cups (473ml) of liquid. Cover and cook over slow heat or in a low oven until meat is tender.

How to broil and grill

- There are two ways to grill pork, directly and indirectly. With direct heat food is placed directly over the heat source. This is ideal for small cuts such as kabobs, tenderloin, burgers and chops. With indirect heat, food is placed on the grill rack away from the coals or burners. This is good for large cuts such as loin roasts, ribs, shoulder and fresh ham.

- Use an instant-read thermometer to determine doneness.

- Trim excess fat to avoid flare-ups while grilling.

- To test the temperature of the coals, hold your hand over them (where the meat would be). If the heat is so intense you must pull away in 3 seconds, the coals are hot. Four seconds indicates medium heat.

- The U.S. Food Code recommends pork be cooked to 145°F (63°C), stuffed pork to 165°F (74°C).

How to roast

- Preheat the oven for at least 10 minutes.

- Allow roasts to rest 10 to 15 minutes before slicing. Cover loosely with a tent made of aluminum foil.

- Place the oven rack in the center of the oven so air can circulate. Be sure to position the rack before turning on the oven.

- Thoroughly preheat the oven before roasting.

Ground pork

- Cook ground pork within 24 hours of thawing. Do not refreeze thawed ground pork.

- Use a meat thermometer to test for doneness of ground pork. Cook on low to medium heat until internal temperature reaches 160°F (71°C).

- Season ground pork before cooking. Recommended seasonings: ginger, cloves, rosemary, chili powder, garlic, oregano, sage and thyme.

Center-Cut Pork Loin, Boneless

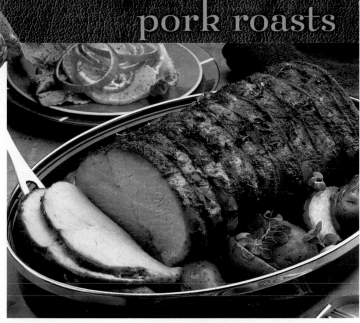

- Roast in a preheated 350°F (177°C) oven and cook for 20 to 25 minutes per pound (.45kg) or to an internal temperature of 145°F (63°C). Let roast rest 10 minutes before carving.

Tip: Pork loin dries out if overcooked. Its flavor and texture improve with brining or soaking in seasoned, salted water for a few hours or up to 24 hours. Flavor with juniper berries, citrus pulp, herbs or honey.

Center-Cut Pork Loin

Nutrition Facts	Amount Per 3-Ounce (85-Gram) Serving, (cooked)			
Calories	180	Total Carbohydrate* 0g 0%	Vitamin A*	0%
Calories from Fat 80		Dietary Fiber* 0g 0%	Vitamin C*	0%
Total Fat*	8g 15%	Sugars 0g	Calcium*	0%
Saturated Fat*	3g 15%	Protein 24g	Iron*	6%
Cholesterol*	70mg 25%	Potassium 361mg	* Percent Daily Values are based on a 2,000 calorie diet. Your daily values may be higher or lower, depending on your calorie needs.	
Sodium*	50mg 2%			

Pork Crown Roast

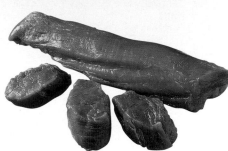

- Cook stuffing separately from the roast. Cook in a preheated 350°F (177°C) oven to an internal temperature of 165°F (74°C) or 20 to 25 minutes per pound (.45kg). Let roast rest 10 minutes before carving. Place stuffing inside the roast.

Tip: Two racks of pork ribs containing 16 to 20 chops are tied in a circle (bones facing up) with space in the center for stuffing to create an impressive crown roast of pork.

Nutrition Facts	Amount Per 3-Ounce (85-Gram) Serving, (cooked)			
Calories	220	Total Carbohydrate* 0g 0%	Vitamin A*	0%
Calories from Fat 120		Dietary Fiber* 0g 0%	Vitamin C*	0%
Total Fat*	13g 20%	Sugars 0g	Calcium*	2%
Saturated Fat*	5g 25%	Protein 23g	Iron*	4%
Cholesterol*	60mg 20%	Potassium 358mg	* Percent Daily Values are based on a 2,000 calorie diet. Your daily values may be higher or lower, depending on your calorie needs.	
Sodium*	40mg 2%			

Pork Tenderloin

- Roast in preheated oven at 450°F (232°C) until the internal temperature reaches 145°F (63°C) or 20 to 30 minutes. Let tenderloin rest for 10 minutes before slicing.
- To grill, butterfly tenderloin. Cook over medium-hot coals for 15 to 25 minutes. Turn once.
- To broil, place butterflied tenderloin 3 to 4 inches (7.62 to 10.16cm) from the heat source and cook for 15 to 25 minutes. Turn once.
- Or, cut into ¾-inch (1.9cm) thick medallions. Sauté for 10 minutes. Turn once.

Tip: Soak dried apricots in white wine for a few hours, then drain. Slash tenderloins end-to-end, and stuff apricots in the slash before roasting. If stuffed, cook to 165°F (74°C).

Nutrition Facts	Amount Per 3-Ounce (85-Gram) Serving, (cooked)			
Calories	140	Total Carbohydrate* 0g 0%	Vitamin A*	0%
Calories from Fat 40		Dietary Fiber* 0g 0%	Vitamin C*	0%
Total Fat*	4g 6%	Sugars 0g	Calcium*	0%
Saturated Fat*	1.5g 8%	Protein 24g	Iron*	6%
Cholesterol*	65mg 20%	Potassium 371mg	* Percent Daily Values are based on a 2,000 calorie diet. Your daily values may be higher or lower, depending on your calorie needs.	
Sodium*	50mg 0%			

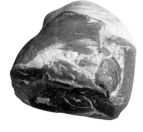

Boston Butt Roast

- To roast, place on rack in a roasting pan. Roast in a preheated 350°F (177°C) oven for 30 to 35 minutes per pound (.45kg) or until the internal temperature reaches 145°F (63°C).
- To braise, brown on all sides in a heavy, lidded casserole. Add 2 cups (473ml) of liquid, cover and cook in a preheated 350°F (177°C) oven for 30 to 35 minutes per pound (.45kg) or to an internal temperature of 155°F to 160°F (68°C to 71°C).

Tip: When braising, be sure the lid of the pot fits snugly so moisture won't escape and the roast won't dry out.

Nutrition Facts	Amount Per 3-Ounce (85-Gram) Serving, (cooked)			
Calories	180	Total Carbohydrate* 0g 0%	Vitamin A*	0%
Calories from Fat 70		Dietary Fiber* 0g 0%	Vitamin C*	0%
Total Fat*	7g 10%	Sugars 0g	Calcium*	0%
Saturated Fat*	2.5g 10%	Protein 26g	Iron*	6%
Cholesterol*	80mg 25%	Potassium 332mg	* Percent Daily Values are based on a 2,000 calorie diet. Your daily values may be higher or lower, depending on your calorie needs.	
Sodium*	55mg 2%			

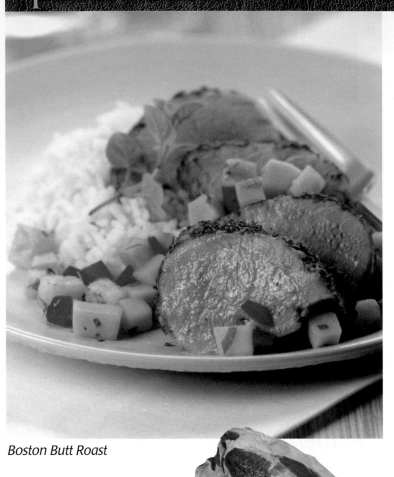

Boston Butt Roast

Sirloin Pork Roast, Bone-In

- Roast in 2 cups (473ml) of liquid, cover and cook in a preheated 350°F (177°C) oven until the internal temperature reaches 145°F (63°C); approximately 25 to 30 minutes per pound (.45kg).

Tip: Before roasting, make an herb paste of garlic, fresh sage and rosemary, pepper and olive oil. Rub and roast.

Picnic Shoulder Arm Roast

- Brown on all sides in a heavy, lidded casserole. Add 2 cups (473ml) of liquid, cover and cook in a preheated 350°F (177°C) oven for 30 to 35 minutes per pound (.45kg) or until the internal temperature reaches 145°F (63°C).

Tip: A picnic roast is best braised or stewed.

Nutrition Facts	Amount Per 3-Ounce (85-Gram) Serving, (cooked)			
Calories	180	Total Carbohydrate* 0g 0%	Vitamin A*	0%
Calories from Fat 80		Dietary Fiber* 0g 0%	Vitamin C*	0%
Total Fat*	9g 15%	Sugars 0g	Calcium*	0%
Saturated Fat*	3g 15%	Protein 24g	Iron*	6%
Cholesterol*	75mg 25%	Potassium 311mg	* Percent Daily Values are based on a 2,000 calorie diet. Your daily values may be higher or lower, depending on your calorie needs.	
Sodium*	55mg 2%			

Nutrition Facts	Amount Per 3-Ounce (85-Gram) Serving, (cooked)			
Calories	270	Total Carbohydrate* 0g 0%	Vitamin A*	0%
Calories from Fat 190		Dietary Fiber* 0g 0%	Vitamin C*	0%
Total Fat*	20g 30%	Sugars 0g	Calcium*	0%
Saturated Fat*	7g 35%	Protein 20g	Iron*	6%
Cholesterol*	80mg 25%	Potassium 276mg	* Percent Daily Values are based on a 2,000 calorie diet. Your daily values may be higher or lower, depending on your calorie needs.	
Sodium*	60mg 2%			

Whole Fresh Leg of Pork

- Have the butcher remove the aitchbone and the skin.
- Place in a roasting pan. Roast in a preheated 350°F (177°C) oven until internal temperature reaches 145°F (63°C), about 22 to 26 minutes per pound (.45kg). Let the roast rest for 30 to 45 minutes before carving.

Tip: Before roasting, cut slits into the meat and insert garlic slices. Season with thyme, oregano and savory to taste. A whole leg makes the perfect centerpiece for family feasts.

Nutrition Facts	Amount Per 3-Ounce (85-Gram) Serving, (cooked)			
Calories 180	Total Carbohydrate* 0g	0%	Vitamin A*	0%
Calories from Fat 80	Dietary Fiber* 0g	0%	Vitamin C*	0%
Total Fat* 8g 10%	Sugars 0g		Calcium*	0%
Saturated Fat* 3g 15%	Protein 25g		Iron*	6%
Cholesterol* 80mg 25%	Potassium 317mg		* Percent Daily Values are based on a 2,000 calorie diet. Your daily values may be higher or lower, depending on your calorie needs.	
Sodium* 55mg 2%				

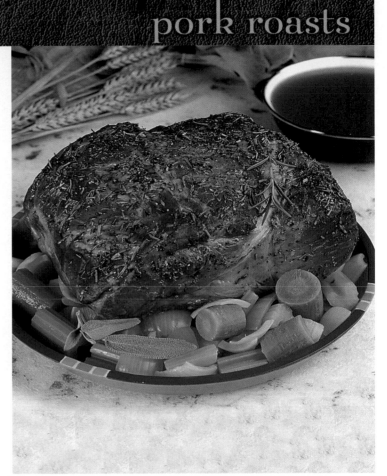

Butt Half Leg of Pork

Butt Half Leg of Pork

- To roast, place in a roasting pan with 2 cups (473ml) of liquid. Roast in a preheated 350°F (177°C) oven for 25 to 35 minutes per pound, (.45kg) or until the internal temperature is 145°F (63°C).

Tip: Thin slices of the leg cut can be used for scallopini or schnitzel. The butt end is more tender than the shank end.

Nutrition Facts	Amount Per 3-Ounce (85-Gram) Serving, (cooked)			
Calories 180	Total Carbohydrate* 0g	0%	Vitamin A*	0%
Calories from Fat 70	Dietary Fiber* 0g	0%	Vitamin C*	0%
Total Fat* 7g 10%	Sugars 0g		Calcium*	0%
Saturated Fat* 2.5g 10%	Protein 26g		Iron*	6%
Cholesterol* 80mg 25%	Potassium 332mg		* Percent Daily Values are based on a 2,000 calorie diet. Your daily values may be higher or lower, depending on your calorie needs.	
Sodium* 55mg 2%				

Shank End Leg of Pork

- Brown on all sides in a heavy, lidded casserole. Add 2 cups (473ml) liquid, cover and cook in a preheated 350°F (177°C) oven for 25 to 35 minutes per pound (.45kg), or until the internal temperature is 145°F (63°C). Let roast rest 10 minutes before carving.

Tip: Smaller bone-in roasts can be either butt half leg or shank end leg.

Nutrition Facts	Amount Per 3-Ounce (85-Gram) Serving, (cooked)			
Calories 180	Total Carbohydrate* 0g	0%	Vitamin A*	0%
Calories from Fat 80	Dietary Fiber* 0g	0%	Vitamin C*	0%
Total Fat* 9g 15%	Sugars 0g		Calcium*	0%
Saturated Fat* 3g 15%	Protein 24g		Iron*	6%
Cholesterol* 80mg 25%	Potassium 306mg		* Percent Daily Values are based on a 2,000 calorie diet. Your daily values may be higher or lower, depending on your calorie needs.	
Sodium* 55mg 2%				

pork chops

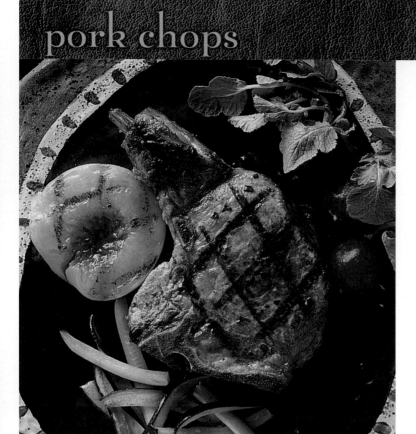

Rib Chop

Loin Chops

- Cook until the internal temperature is 145°F (63°C). Let rest for 5 minutes before serving.
- Grill ¾-inch-thick (1.9cm) chops over medium-hot coals for 6 to 8 minutes.
- Broil ¾-inch-thick (1.9cm) chops 3 to 4 inches (7.62 to 10.16cm) from the heat source for 6 to 8 minutes.
- Sauté ¾-inch-thick (1.9cm) chops in 2 tablespoons (30ml) of oil over medium-high heat for 6 to 10 minutes.

Tip: Loin chops have a T-bone shape. Buy thick chops so they don't dry out.

Nutrition Facts	Amount Per 3-Ounce (85-Gram) Serving, (cooked)				
Calories	170	Total Carbohydrate* 0g 0%		Vitamin A*	0%
Calories from Fat	60	Dietary Fiber* 0g 0%		Vitamin C*	0%
Total Fat*	7g 10%	Sugars	0g	Calcium*	2%
Saturated Fat*	2.5g 10%	Protein	26g	Iron*	4%
Cholesterol*	70mg 25%	Potassium	357mg	* Percent Daily Values are based on a 2,000 calorie diet. Your daily values may be higher or lower, depending on your calorie needs.	
Sodium*	55mg 2%				

Rib Chops

- Cook until the internal temperature is 145°F (63°C). Let chops rest 5 minutes before serving.
- Grill ¾-inch-thick (1.9cm) chops over medium-hot coals for 6 to 8 minutes. Turn once.
- Broil ¾-inch-thick (1.9cm) chops 3 to 4 inches (7.62 to 10.16cm) from the heat source for 6 to 8 minutes. Turn once.
- Sauté ¾-inch-thick (1.9cm) chops in 2 tablespoons (30ml) oil over medium-high heat for 6 to 10 minutes. Turn once.

Tip: Sauté in sesame oil for a rich, nutty flavor.

Sirloin Chops, Boneless

- Brown ¾-inch-thick (1.9cm) sirloin boneless chops on both sides in a heavy, lidded casserole. Add ½ to 2 cups (118 to 473ml) of liquid, cover and cook for 20 minutes, or until the internal temperature is 145°F (63°C). Let rest 5 minutes before serving.

Tip: Looking to reduce your sodium intake? Try a salt-free lemon-herb seasoning for plenty of flavor without the sodium.

Nutrition Facts	Amount Per 3-Ounce (85-Gram) Serving, (cooked)				
Calories	190	Total Carbohydrate* 0g 0%		Vitamin A*	0%
Calories from Fat	80	Dietary Fiber* 0g 0%		Vitamin C*	0%
Total Fat*	8g 15%	Sugars	0g	Calcium*	2%
Saturated Fat*	3g 15%	Protein	26g	Iron*	4%
Cholesterol*	70mg 25%	Potassium	357mg	* Percent Daily Values are based on a 2,000 calorie diet. Your daily values may be higher or lower, depending on your calorie needs.	
Sodium*	55mg 2%				

Nutrition Facts	Amount Per 3-Ounce (85-Gram) Serving, (cooked)				
Calories	170	Total Carbohydrate* 0g 0%		Vitamin A*	0%
Calories from Fat	60	Dietary Fiber* 0g 0%		Vitamin C*	0%
Total Fat*	7g 10%	Sugars	0g	Calcium*	2%
Saturated Fat*	2.5g 10%	Protein	26g	Iron*	4%
Cholesterol*	70mg 25%	Potassium	357mg	* Percent Daily Values are based on a 2,000 calorie diet. Your daily values may be higher or lower, depending on your calorie needs.	
Sodium*	55mg 2%				

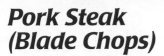

Pork Steak (Blade Chops)

- Cook until the internal temperature reaches 145°F (63°C).
- Grill ¾-inch-thick (1.9cm) blade chops over medium-hot coals for 6 to 8 minutes. Turn once. Let rest 5 minutes before serving.
- Brown a ¾-inch-thick (1.9cm) blade chop on both sides. Add ½ to 2 cups (118 to 473ml) of liquid. Cover tightly, and simmer for 20 minutes. Let rest 5 minutes before serving.

Tip: Sprinkling with ginger and braising in orange juice brings out the sweet succulence of pork.

Nutrition Facts	Amount Per 3-Ounce (85-Gram) Serving, (cooked)				
Calories	190	Total Carbohydrate*	0g	0%	Vitamin A*	0%
Calories from Fat 100		Dietary Fiber*	0g	0%	Vitamin C*	0%
Total Fat*	11g 15%	Sugars	0g		Calcium*	2%
Saturated Fat*	4g 20%	Protein	23g		Iron*	8%
Cholesterol*	80mg 25%	Potassium	292mg		* Percent Daily Values are based on a 2,000 calorie diet. Your daily values may be higher or lower, depending on your calorie needs.
Sodium*	65mg 2%				

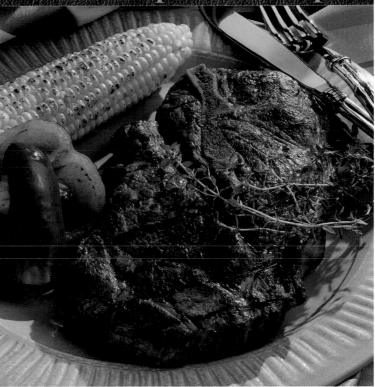

Pork Steak

Smoked Chops

- Place ¾-inch-thick (1.9cm) smoked chops in a roasting pan. Add 1 cup (237ml) of liquid, cover and cook in a preheated 350°F (177°C) oven for 10 to 20 minutes or until warm.

Tip: Try serving with an easy sauce of apple cider, fresh sage, vinegar and Dijon mustard.

Nutrition Facts	Amount Per 3-Ounce (85-Gram) Serving, (cooked)				
Calories	240	Total Carbohydrate*	0g	0%	Vitamin A*	0%
Calories from Fat 160		Dietary Fiber*	0g	0%	Vitamin C*	0%
Total Fat*	18g 28%	Sugars	0g		Calcium*	0%
Saturated Fat*	7g 35%	Protein	17g		Iron*	4%
Cholesterol*	50mg 17%	Potassium	219mg		* Percent Daily Values are based on a 2,000 calorie diet. Your daily values may be higher or lower, depending on your calorie needs.
Sodium*	910mg 38%				

Pork Chops, Center-Cut

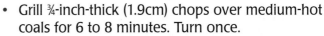

- Cook until the internal temperature reaches 145°F (63°C). Let chops rest 5 minutes before serving.
- Grill ¾-inch-thick (1.9cm) chops over medium-hot coals for 6 to 8 minutes. Turn once.
- Broil ¾-inch-thick (1.9cm) chops 3 to 4 inches (7.62 to 10.16cm) from the heat 6 to 8 minutes. Turn once.
- Sauté ¾-inch-thick (1.9cm) chops in 2 tablespoons (30ml) of oil over medium-high heat for 6 to 10 minutes. Turn once.

Tip: Combine butter, white wine, chicken broth and shallots for a simple sauce.

Nutrition Facts	Amount Per 3-Ounce (85-Gram) Serving, (cooked)				
Calories	170	Total Carbohydrate*	0g	0%	Vitamin A*	0%
Calories from Fat 60		Dietary Fiber*	0g	0%	Vitamin C*	0%
Total Fat*	7g 10%	Sugars	0g		Calcium*	2%
Saturated Fat*	2.5g 15%	Protein	26g		Iron*	4%
Cholesterol*	70mg 25%	Potassium	319mg		* Percent Daily Values are based on a 2,000 calorie diet. Your daily values may be higher or lower, depending on your calorie needs.
Sodium*	50mg 2%				

Pork Spareribs

- Place on a rack in a roasting pan. Cook for 1½ to 2 hours in a preheated 350°F (177°C) oven. Add sauce the last half-hour. Cook to an internal temperature of 145°F (63°C).

Tip: Baste while roasting. Plan on 2 to 3 servings per slab.

Nutrition Facts	Amount Per 3-Ounce (85-Gram) Serving, (cooked)		
Calories 340	Total Carbohydrate* 0g 0%	Vitamin A*	0%
Calories from Fat 240	Dietary Fiber* 0g 0%	Vitamin C*	0%
Total Fat* 26g 40%	Sugars 0g	Calcium*	4%
Saturated Fat* 9g 45%	Protein 25g	Iron*	8%
Cholesterol* 105mg 35%	Potassium 272mg	* Percent Daily Values are based on a 2,000 calorie diet. Your daily values may be higher or lower, depending on your calorie needs.	
Sodium* 80mg 4%			

Pork Baby Back Ribs

- Place on a rack in a roasting pan. Cook for 1½ to 2 hours in a preheated 350°F (177°C) oven. Add sauce the last half-hour. Internal temperature should be 145°F (63°C).

Tip: Add sugar-based barbecue sauces after grilling.

Nutrition Facts	Amount Per 3-Ounce (85-Gram) Serving, (cooked)		
Calories 310	Total Carbohydrate* 0g 0%	Vitamin A*	0%
Calories from Fat 230	Dietary Fiber* 0g 0%	Vitamin C*	0%
Total Fat* 25g 40%	Sugars 0g	Calcium*	4%
Saturated Fat* 9g 45%	Protein 21g	Iron*	6%
Cholesterol* 100mg 35%	Potassium 268mg	* Percent Daily Values are based on a 2,000 calorie diet. Your daily values may be higher or lower, depending on your calorie needs.	
Sodium* 85mg 4%			

Pork Country-Style Ribs, Boneless

- Brown on all sides in a heavy, lidded casserole. Add 1 cup (237ml) of wine or other liquid. Bring to a boil. Cover and simmer for 2 hours, or until the internal temperature is 145°F (63°C).
- Roast in a preheated 350°F (177°C) oven for 2 hours, or until the internal temperature is 145°F (63°C).

Tip: From the blade end of the loin, these inexpensive ribs are good slowly grilled or braised. Crisp under the broiler if desired.

Nutrition Facts	Amount Per 3-Ounce (85-Gram) Serving, (cooked)		
Calories 210	Total Carbohydrate* 0g 0%	Vitamin A*	0%
Calories from Fat 120	Dietary Fiber* 0g 0%	Vitamin C*	0%
Total Fat* 13g 20%	Sugars 0g	Calcium*	2%
Saturated Fat* 4.5g 25%	Protein 23g	Iron*	6%
Cholesterol* 80mg 25%	Potassium 297mg	* Percent Daily Values are based on a 2,000 calorie diet. Your daily values may be higher or lower, depending on your calorie needs.	
Sodium* 25mg 0%			

Pork Country-Style Ribs

- Roast in a preheated 350°F (177°C) oven, loosely covered with aluminum foil for 1 hour. Turn ribs once at 30 minutes. Pour 1 cup (237ml) of sweet vermouth on the ribs. Continue to cook for another hour, basting every 10 minutes. Total cooking time is 2 hours. Internal temperature should be 145°F (63°C). Let rest 5 minutes before serving.
- Or, brown on all sides in a heavy, lidded casserole. Add 2 cups (473ml) of liquid. Cover and cook in a preheated 350°F (177°C) oven for 2 hours or until the internal temperature is 145°F (63°C).

Tip: Use 3 to 4 tablespoons (44.34 to 59.12ml) of spice rub per slab.

Nutrition Facts	Amount Per 3-Ounce (85-Gram) Serving, (cooked)		
Calories 250	Total Carbohydrate* 0g 0%	Vitamin A*	0%
Calories from Fat 160	Dietary Fiber* 0g 0%	Vitamin C*	0%
Total Fat* 18g 28%	Sugars 0g	Calcium*	2%
Saturated Fat* 7g 35%	Protein 20g	Iron*	6%
Cholesterol* 75mg 25%	Potassium 279mg	* Percent Daily Values are based on a 2,000 calorie diet. Your daily values may be higher or lower, depending on your calorie needs.	
Sodium* 50mg 2%			

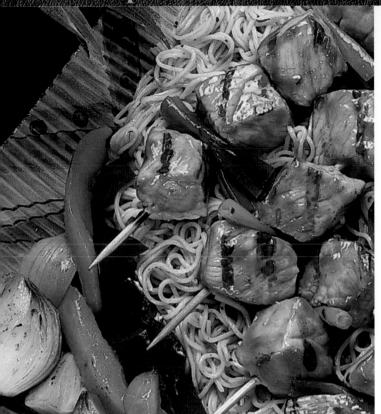

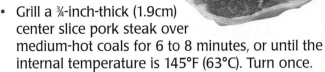

Pork Leg Steak, Center Slice

- Grill a ¾-inch-thick (1.9cm) center slice pork steak over medium-hot coals for 6 to 8 minutes, or until the internal temperature is 145°F (63°C). Turn once.
- Sauté a ¾-inch-thick (1.9cm) center slice pork steak in 2 tablespoons (30ml) of oil over medium-high heat for 6 to 10 minutes, or until the internal temperature is 145°F (63°C). Turn once.

Tip: Pork steaks are best when marinated and grilled or pan-fried or pounded into pork cutlets with the bone removed.

Nutrition Facts		Amount Per 3-Ounce (85-Gram) Serving, (cooked)				
Calories	180	Total Carbohydrate*	0g	0%	Vitamin A*	0%
Calories from Fat	70	Dietary Fiber*	0g	0%	Vitamin C*	0%
Total Fat*	7g 10%	Sugars		0g	Calcium*	0%
Saturated Fat*	2.5g 10%	Protein		26g	Iron*	6%
Cholesterol*	80mg 25%	Potassium		332mg	* Percent Daily Values are based on a 2,000 calorie diet. Your daily values may be higher or lower, depending on your calorie needs.	
Sodium*	55mg 2%					

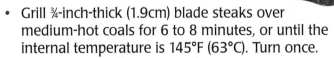

Pork Blade Steak

Pork Blade Steak

- Grill ¾-inch-thick (1.9cm) blade steaks over medium-hot coals for 6 to 8 minutes, or until the internal temperature is 145°F (63°C). Turn once.
- Brown ¾-inch-thick (1.9cm) blade steaks on both sides. Add 1 cup (237ml) of liquid, cover and cook over low heat for 20 minutes, or until the internal temperature is 145°F (63°C).

Tip: Mustard is a natural flavor pairing with the sweet taste of pork; use sparingly as a rub before cooking, and try different kinds, such as raspberry or honey mustard.

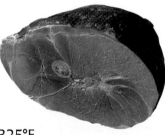

Ham

- Fully cooked ham is ready to serve.
- Roast in a preheated 325°F (163°C) oven for 20 minutes per pound (.45kg).
- To grill, use indirect heat in a covered grill. When ham reaches an internal temperature of 130°F (54°C), add glaze and transfer to a preheated 425°F (218°C) oven. Roast for 20 minutes.

Tip: Try adding cloves, fruit juice, jam or marmalade to marinades.

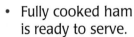
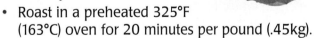

Nutrition Facts		Amount Per 3-Ounce (85-Gram) Serving, (cooked)				
Calories	220	Total Carbohydrate*	0g	0%	Vitamin A*	0%
Calories from Fat	130	Dietary Fiber*	0g	0%	Vitamin C*	0%
Total Fat*	14g 20%	Sugars		0g	Calcium*	4%
Saturated Fat*	5g 25%	Protein		22g	Iron*	6%
Cholesterol*	80mg 25%	Potassium		277mg	* Percent Daily Values are based on a 2,000 calorie diet. Your daily values may be higher or lower, depending on your calorie needs.	
Sodium*	60mg 2%					

Nutrition Facts		Amount Per 3-Ounce (85-Gram) Serving, (cooked)				
Calories	130	Total Carbohydrate*	0g	0%	Vitamin A*	0%
Calories from Fat	45	Dietary Fiber*	0g	0%	Vitamin C*	0%
Total Fat*	4.5g 8%	Sugars		0g	Calcium*	0%
Saturated Fat*	1.5g 8%	Protein		21g	Iron*	4%
Cholesterol*	45mg 15%	Potassium		269mg	* Percent Daily Values are based on a 2,000 calorie diet. Your daily values may be higher or lower, depending on your calorie needs.	
Sodium*	1130mg 45%					

Pork Neck Bones

- To make a delicious stock, brown in a preheated 350°F (177°C) oven until golden brown. Add to 3 quarts (2.83l) of cold water. Bring to a boil. Reduce heat and simmer for 4 hours. Add vegetables in the last hour. Strain.

Tip: Pork neck bones also add hearty flavor to beans, lentils, pea soup and cabbage.

Nutrition Facts	Amount Per 3-Ounce (85-Gram) Serving, (cooked)			
Calories	180	Total Carbohydrate* 0g 0%	Vitamin A* 0%
Calories from Fat 70		Dietary Fiber* 0g 0%	Vitamin C* 0%
Total Fat*	8g 12%	Sugars 0g	Calcium* 0%
Saturated Fat*	3g 13%	Protein 24g	Iron* 6%
Cholesterol*	70mg 23%	Potassium 296mg	* Percent Daily Values are based on a 2,000 calorie diet. Your daily values may be higher or lower, depending on your calorie needs.
Sodium*	570mg 24%		

Pigs' Tails

- Brown tails in a heavy, lidded casserole. Add 3 cups (710ml) liquid. Cover and cook for 1½ hours. Remove cover. Simmer for 1 hour, or until the liquid is reduced by one-half.

Tip: Without much meat, pigs' tails add flavor to slow-cooked dishes.

Nutrition Facts	Amount Per 3-Ounce (85-Gram) Serving, (cooked)			
Calories	340	Total Carbohydrate* 0g 0%	Vitamin A* 0%
Calories from Fat 280		Dietary Fiber* 0g 0%	Vitamin C* 0%
Total Fat*	30g 45%	Sugars 0g	Calcium* 0%
Saturated Fat*	11g 50%	Protein 14g	Iron* 4%
Cholesterol*	110mg 35%	Potassium 133mg	* Percent Daily Values are based on a 2,000 calorie diet. Your daily values may be higher or lower, depending on your calorie needs.
Sodium*	20mg 0%		

Pigs' Feet

- Thoroughly wash whole pigs' feet. Place in pot. Add enough water to cover them. Add vegetables such as okra or root vegetables. Bring to a boil. Reduce heat and simmer for 2½ to 3 hours.
- Internal temperature should be 145°F (63°C).

Tip: Mostly bone, fat and skin, pigs' feet add flavor and substance to some slow-cooked Caribbean dishes.

Nutrition Facts	Amount Per 3-Ounce (85-Gram) Serving, (cooked)			
Calories	160	Total Carbohydrate* 0g 0%	Vitamin A* 0%
Calories from Fat 100		Dietary Fiber* 0g 0%	Vitamin C* 0%
Total Fat*	11g 15%	Sugars 0g	Calcium* 4%
Saturated Fat*	3.5g 20%	Protein 16g	Iron* 2%
Cholesterol*	85mg 30%	Potassium 124mg	* Percent Daily Values are based on a 2,000 calorie diet. Your daily values may be higher or lower, depending on your calorie needs.
Sodium*	25mg 0%		

Pork Hocks

- Place hocks (preferably smoked ham hocks) in a large pot. Add enough water to cover. Bring water to a boil, then reduce heat to low. Simmer for 2 hours. Add 4 10-ounce (284g) packages of frozen lima beans and cook until the beans are tender – 10 minutes.

Tip: Ham hocks are delicious cooked with lima, red, navy beans or sauerkraut.

Nutrition Facts	Amount Per 3-Ounce (85-Gram) Serving, (cooked)			
Calories	280	Total Carbohydrate* 0g 0%	Vitamin A* 0%
Calories from Fat 180		Dietary Fiber* 0g 0%	Vitamin C* 0%
Total Fat*	20g 31%	Sugars 0g	Calcium* 2%
Saturated Fat*	7g 35%	Protein 24g	Iron* 8%
Cholesterol*	95mg 32%	Potassium 314mg	* Percent Daily Values are based on a 2,000 calorie diet. Your daily values may be higher or lower, depending on your calorie needs.
Sodium*	75mg 3%		

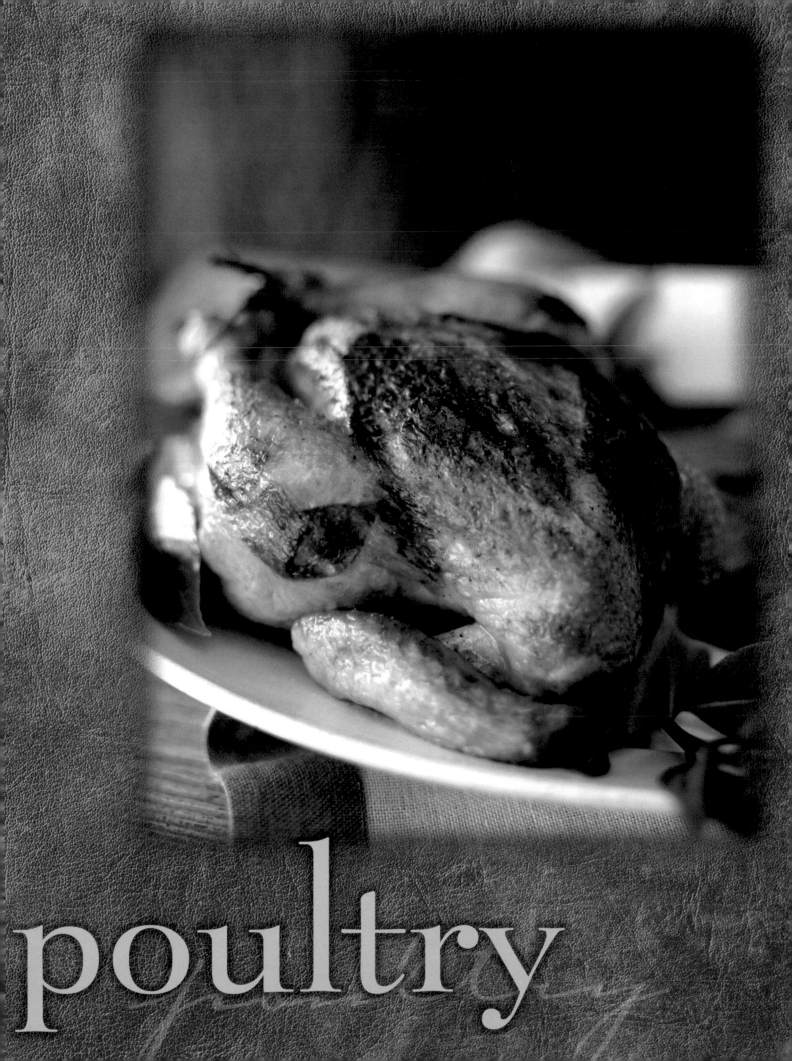

poultry

What makes white meat "white?"

Muscle becomes red or "dark meat" when the protein myosin absorbs a lot of oxygen. This happens when the muscles are heavily worked. The breast of a flightless chicken is not exercised, so it remains "white."

Why is a ground turkey hamburger drier than a beef hamburger?

Beef contains more fat than turkey. To make a juicy turkey burger, add some stock, an egg or water-rich vegetables such as spinach to ground turkey. Cook as normal.

What is a tom turkey?

Tom turkeys are male and can weigh up to 25 pounds (11.36kg). The female turkey is called a hen. Hens weigh 10 to 18 pounds (4.55 to 8.18kg).

How fresh is a "fresh" turkey?

Fresh turkeys can be kept at 26°F (-3°C) for a few weeks and still be considered fresh. Fresh turkeys are considered to be tastier and more tender.

What are giblets?

Giblets are the heart, gizzard and liver of a bird.

What is a Rock Cornish game hen?

Rock Cornish game hens are simply very young chickens. They weigh about 1¼ pounds (.57kg). Generally, you should serve one per person.

How does poultry compare to beef nutritionally?

Cooked, a trimmed piece of lean beef has three times the fat of a light-meat skinless piece of chicken (9 grams vs. 3 grams). Chicken also provides a good source of niacin and protein. Turkey is the leanest of all meats with less than 1 gram of fat and 135 calories (536.62kJ) in a 3.5-ounce (99g) serving.

How is chicken graded?

Chicken is graded by the United States Department of Agriculture and the Canadian Food Inspection Agency on appearance, not on fat content. *Grade A* means the chicken is well-formed, free of feathers and has a layer of fat with unblemished skin. The same is true of turkey.

SELECTION

Chicken

- Check the "sell-by" date on the label. Don't buy if date has passed.
- Whole chickens should have a regular shape with a plump breast. Skin should be unblemished.
- When buying parts look for packages without any pink-tinged liquid.

Turkey

- Turkeys are now available fresh and frozen all year long. Fresh turkey must be cooked within 2 days of the "sell-by" date.
- Frozen turkeys should be rock hard and free of ice crystals and freezer burn. Turkey parts should be moist and pink. The skin should be creamy white, not bluish.

Duck

- Ninety percent of all duck sold is frozen. If you find a fresh duck, look for white, not yellow, skin that is free of feathers and blemishes.

STORAGE

- Keep fresh poultry in the coldest part of the refrigerator and use within 2 days.

HANDLING

- Poultry should be handled carefully to avoid the spreading of bacteria. Always wash utensils, cutting boards, dishes and hands with hot soapy water after working with raw poultry.
- Rinse the bird or its parts under cold running water. Be sure to rinse the cavity as well. Remove excess deposits of fat.
- Never thaw poultry at room temperature; defrost in the refrigerator.

POULTRY CUT	ROAST	GRILL/BROIL	STIR-FRY	SAUTÉ	BRAISE	DEEP-FRY
Chicken, Whole Roasting	X	Indirect heat in a covered grill				
Chicken Fryer	X	X			X	X
Chicken Breast	X	X			X	X
Chicken Drumsticks	X	X			X	X
Chicken Thighs	X	X			X	X
Chicken Wings	X	X			X	X
Chicken Thighs, Boneless	X	X	X	X	X	X
Chicken Breast, Boneless	X	X	X	X	X	X
Chicken Stir-Fry			X			
Cornish Game Hen	X	X				
Chicken, Stewing					X	
Chicken Fryer Leg Quarter	X	X			X	X
Duck	X	X (Boneless)		X (Boneless Breasts)	X (Pieces)	
Turkey, Whole	X	Indirect heat in a covered grill				X
Turkey Breast	X	Indirect heat in a covered grill				X
Turkey Drumsticks	X	Indirect heat in a covered grill			X	
Turkey Thighs		X			X	
Turkey Wings					X	
Turkey Breast Roast, Boneless	X	Indirect heat in a covered grill				
Turkey Tenderloins		X	X		X	
Turkey Cutlets		X	X	X		X
Turkey, Ground		X		X		

How to broil and grill

- Broil on rack 6 inches (15.24cm) from heat. Always broil the bone side first.

- Turn meat at least once.

- Always leave the skin on during cooking. The skin seals in the juices, making the meat very tender. Cook until skin is crispy.

- Poultry is done when the juices run clear and the meat is no longer pink. For large birds, use a meat thermometer – it should register 180°F (82°C) in the thigh and 165°F to 170°F (74°C to 77°C) for the breast.

- Boneless birds cook in about half the time of bone-in birds.

How to roast

- Preheat the oven for at least 10 minutes.

- Roast breast with skin side up.

- Use an instant-read thermometer. Insert halfway into roast, making sure not to touch bone.

- Always allow poultry to rest 10 to 15 minutes after cooking before slicing. Cover loosely with a tent of aluminum foil.

- Allow an extra 20 minutes if the bird is stuffed. Stuffing should register at 165°F (74°C).

- For more tender meat and to minimize shrinkage from loss of moisture, use a moderately slow oven temperature of 325°F (163°C).

How to sauté

- Do not add water or cover.

- Use a small amount of oil or butter.

- Cook quickly over medium-high heat, with sufficient moisture to prevent tough poultry.

- Remember: boneless, skinless poultry is easy to overcook, so watch carefully and keep moist.

- White meat cooks faster than dark meat, so be sure to separate the parts. Add white meat approximately 5 minutes after the dark meat.

Marinating

- The best way to marinate poultry is to place it in a resealable plastic bag with the marinade and refrigerate. Be sure to squeeze out as much air as possible and turn the bag several times.

- Whole chickens can take up to 12 hours to marinate; while boneless, skinless pieces take a quarter of that time.

- Always refrigerate poultry while it is marinating. Letting them stand at room temperature invites bacteria.

Whole Roasting Chicken

- Rub a roasting chicken with herbs. Place on a rack in a shallow pan. Roast in preheated oven at 350°F (177°C) for 20 minutes per pound (.45kg) plus 15 minutes. Internal temperature of the thigh should read 180°F (82°C). If bird is stuffed, allow an extra 20 minutes. Let chicken rest 10 minutes before carving.

Tip: To reduce fat, cook whole birds on a rack.

Nutrition Facts			Amount Per 3-Ounce (85-Gram) Serving, (cooked)		
Calories	190		Total Carbohydrate* 0g 0%	Vitamin A*	2%
Calories from Fat 100			Dietary Fiber* 0g 0%	Vitamin C*	0%
Total Fat*	11g	17%	Sugars 0g	Calcium*	2%
Saturated Fat*	3g	15%	Protein 20g	Iron*	6%
Cholesterol*	65mg	22%	Potassium 179mg	* Percent Daily Values are based on a 2,000 calorie diet. Your daily values may be higher or lower, depending on your calorie needs.	
Sodium*	60mg	3%			

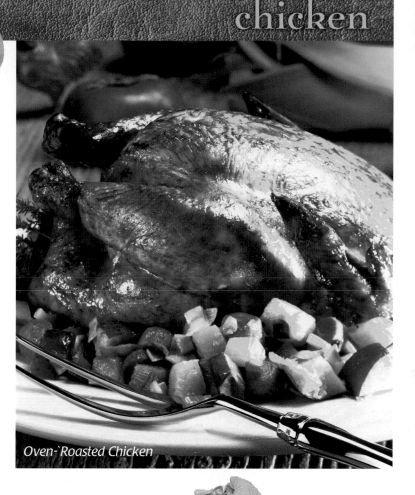

Oven-`Roasted Chicken

Chicken Fryer

- Fryers can be roasted whole or cut into parts and braised, fried or broiled.

- Place an herb-seasoned fryer on a rack in a shallow pan. Roast in a preheated 350°F (177°C) oven for 20 minutes per pound (.45kg) plus 15 minutes. Internal temperature of the thigh should read 180°F (82°C). If bird is stuffed, allow an extra 20 minutes. Let chicken rest for 10 minutes before carving.

Tip: To fry, mix milk and egg for wash. Dip fryer pieces in mixture to coat. Dredge in seasoned flour.

Nutrition Facts			Amount Per 3-Ounce (85-Gram) Serving, (cooked)		
Calories	200		Total Carbohydrate* 0g 0%	Vitamin A*	2%
Calories from Fat 100			Dietary Fiber* 0g 0%	Vitamin C*	0%
Total Fat*	12g	18%	Sugars 0g	Calcium*	2%
Saturated Fat*	3g	15%	Protein 23g	Iron*	6%
Cholesterol*	75mg	25%	Potassium 190mg	* Percent Daily Values are based on a 2,000 calorie diet. Your daily values may be higher or lower, depending on your calorie needs.	
Sodium*	70mg	3%			

Chicken Breast

- Chicken breasts can be roasted, grilled, braised or fried.

- To roast, dredge breasts in flour. Cook in a preheated 350°F (177°C) oven for 30 to 40 minutes or until internal temperature reaches 165°F (74°C).

- Grill or broil breasts for 10 to 15 minutes per side until internal temperature reaches 165°F (74°C).

Tip: Marinate chicken breasts in bottled Italian dressing before cooking for an easy and flavorful main course. Discard marinade after use.

Nutrition Facts			Amount Per 3-Ounce (85-Gram) Serving, (cooked)		
Calories	170		Total Carbohydrate* 0g 0%	Vitamin A*	2%
Calories from Fat 60			Dietary Fiber* 0g 0%	Vitamin C*	0%
Total Fat*	7g	11%	Sugars 0g	Calcium*	2%
Saturated Fat*	2g	10%	Protein 25g	Iron*	6%
Cholesterol*	70mg	23%	Potassium 210mg	* Percent Daily Values are based on a 2,000 calorie diet. Your daily values may be higher or lower, depending on your calorie needs.	
Sodium*	60mg	3%			

Chicken Thighs

- Chicken thighs can be grilled, broiled, roasted, braised or fried.
- To grill or broil, cook 10 to 15 minutes per side or until internal temperature reaches 165°F (74°C).
- To roast, cook in a preheated 350°F (177°C) oven for 40 to 50 minutes. Thighs are done when juices run clear; or when internal temperature reaches 165°F (74°C).

Tip: Thaw frozen poultry completely before cooking. To test doneness, pierce the thigh with a skewer; juices should be clear, not pink.

Nutrition Facts	Amount Per 3-Ounce (85-Gram) Serving, (cooked)				
Calories	210	Total Carbohydrate*	0g 0%	Vitamin A*	2%
Calories from Fat 120		Dietary Fiber*	0g 0%	Vitamin C*	0%
Total Fat*	13g 20%	Sugars	0g	Calcium*	2%
Saturated Fat*	3.5g 18%	Protein	21g	Iron*	6%
Cholesterol*	80mg 27%	Potassium	189mg	* Percent Daily Values are based on a 2,000 calorie diet. Your daily values may be higher or lower, depending on your calorie needs.	
Sodium*	70mg 3%				

Chicken Drumsticks

- Drumsticks can be roasted, grilled, broiled, braised or deep-fried.
- To roast, cook in a preheated 350°F (177°C) oven for 35 to 45 minutes or until internal temperature reaches 165°F (74°C).
- To broil or grill, cook drumsticks 10 to 15 minutes per side or until juices run clear; to an internal temperature of 165°F (74°C).

Tip: Before breading drumsticks, roll in plain low-fat yogurt for moist, flavorful results.

Nutrition Facts	Amount Per 3-Ounce (85-Gram) Serving, (cooked)				
Calories	150	Total Carbohydrate*	0g 0%	Vitamin A*	0%
Calories from Fat 45		Dietary Fiber*	0g 0%	Vitamin C*	0%
Total Fat*	5g 8%	Sugars	0g	Calcium*	2%
Saturated Fat*	1.5g 8%	Protein	24g	Iron*	6%
Cholesterol*	80mg 27%	Potassium	209mg	* Percent Daily Values are based on a 2,000 calorie diet. Your daily values may be higher or lower, depending on your calorie needs.	
Sodium*	80mg 3%				

Chicken Wings

- Chicken wings can be grilled, broiled, roasted or fried.
- To get them really crispy, dredge them in flour with garlic powder. Roast in a preheated 350°F (177°C) oven for 30 to 40 minutes or to an internal temperature 165°F (74°C).

Tip: Accompany spicy chicken wings with palate-cooling celery sticks and ranch dressing instead of blue cheese for a refreshing change of taste.

Nutrition Facts	Amount Per 3-Ounce (85-Gram) Serving, (cooked)				
Calories	130	Total Carbohydrate*	0g 0%	Vitamin A*	0%
Calories from Fat 45		Dietary Fiber*	0g 0%	Vitamin C*	0%
Total Fat*	5g 8%	Sugars	0g	Calcium*	2%
Saturated Fat*	1.5g 8%	Protein	23g	Iron*	4%
Cholesterol*	55mg 18%	Potassium	132mg	* Percent Daily Values are based on a 2,000 calorie diet. Your daily values may be higher or lower, depending on your calorie needs.	
Sodium*	60mg 3%				

Chicken Thighs, Boneless

- Broil or grill for 10 to 12 minutes per side or to an internal temperature of 160°F (71°C).
- Roast in a preheated 350°F (177°C) oven for 40 to 45 minutes or to an internal temperature of 165°F (74°C).
- Or, brown and braise for 20 to 25 minutes. Thighs are done when juices run clear.

Tip: To debone, slit lengthwise through meat.

Nutrition Facts	Amount Per 3-Ounce (85-Gram) Serving, (cooked)				
Calories	180	Total Carbohydrate*	0g 0%	Vitamin A*	2%
Calories from Fat	80	Dietary Fiber*	0g 0%	Vitamin C*	0%
Total Fat*	9g 14%	Sugars	0g	Calcium*	2%
Saturated Fat*	3g 13%	Protein	22g	Iron*	6%
Cholesterol*	80mg 27%	Potassium	202mg	* Percent Daily Values are based on a 2,000 calorie diet. Your daily values may be higher or lower, depending on your calorie needs.	
Sodium*	75mg 3%				

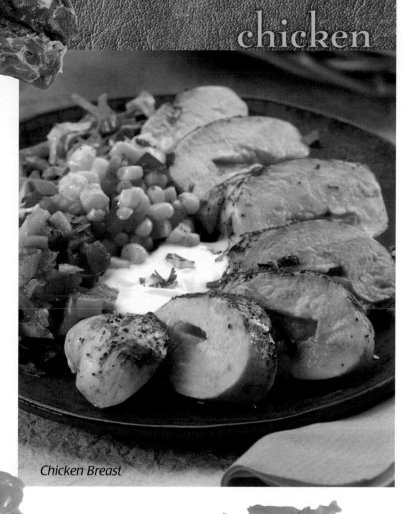

Chicken Breast

Chicken Breast, Boneless

- To sauté, heat a small amount of butter or oil over medium-high heat. Cook for 15 to 20 minutes, turning once. If they have been flattened with a mallet, they only need 10 to 15 minutes to cook.
- To grill, cook over medium-hot coals for 6 to 8 minutes per side or to an internal temperature of 165°F (74°C). Turn once.
- Broil 9 inches (22.86cm) from heat source for 5 to 6 minutes per side. Turn once.
- Bake in a preheated 350°F (177°C) oven for 35 minutes.

Tip: These make a great substitute for veal cutlets in recipes such as veal piccata; just pound breasts to ¼-inch thick (.64cm) and increase cooking time.

Chicken Stir-Fry

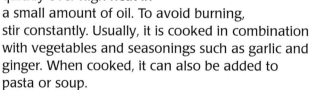

- Chicken stir-fry is cut into narrow strips from white breast meat. It is cooked quickly over high heat in a small amount of oil. To avoid burning, stir constantly. Usually, it is cooked in combination with vegetables and seasonings such as garlic and ginger. When cooked, it can also be added to pasta or soup.

Tip: Carefully coat preheated wok with 1 tablespoon (15ml) of oil. Use a folding motion to quickly stir ingredients.

Nutrition Facts	Amount Per 3-Ounce (85-Gram) Serving, (cooked)				
Calories	140	Total Carbohydrate*	0g 0%	Vitamin A*	0%
Calories from Fat	25	Dietary Fiber*	0g 0%	Vitamin C*	0%
Total Fat*	3g 5%	Sugars	0g	Calcium*	2%
Saturated Fat*	1g 5%	Protein	26g	Iron*	4%
Cholesterol*	70mg 23%	Potassium	218mg	* Percent Daily Values are based on a 2,000 calorie diet. Your daily values may be higher or lower, depending on your calorie needs.	
Sodium*	65mg 3%				

Nutrition Facts	Amount Per 3-Ounce (85-Gram) Serving, (cooked)				
Calories	200	Total Carbohydrate*	0g 0%	Vitamin A*	0%
Calories from Fat	90	Dietary Fiber*	0g 0%	Vitamin C*	0%
Total Fat*	10g 15%	Sugars	0g	Calcium*	2%
Saturated Fat*	1.5g 8%	Protein	26g	Iron*	4%
Cholesterol*	70mg 23%	Potassium	218mg	* Percent Daily Values are based on a 2,000 calorie diet. Your daily values may be higher or lower, depending on your calorie needs.	
Sodium*	65mg 3%				

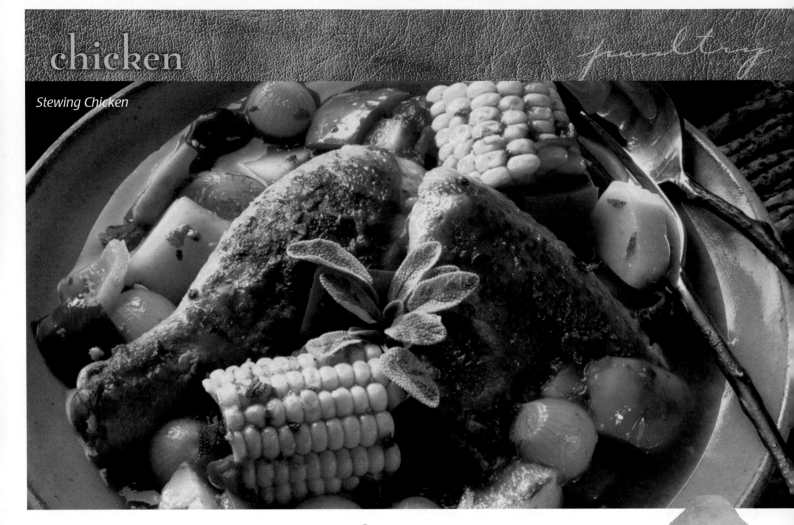

Stewing Chicken

Stewing Chicken

- A true stewing hen is a mature hen and requires 1 to 2 hours of gentle cooking. Any chicken can be stewed, however. Clean the bird; place in a large, heavy kettle. Add liquid to nearly cover the bird, and some seasonings. Cover and simmer until tender. With a younger bird, this could take as little as 45 minutes.

Tip: For richer flavor, stew in low-sodium chicken broth or wine instead of water.

Nutrition Facts	Amount Per 3-Ounce (85-Gram) Serving, (cooked)		
Calories 240	Total Carbohydrate* 0g 0%	Vitamin A*	2%
Calories from Fat 140	Dietary Fiber* 0g 0%	Vitamin C*	0%
Total Fat* 16g 25%	Sugars 0g	Calcium*	2%
Saturated Fat* 5g 23%	Protein 23g	Iron*	6%
Cholesterol* 65mg 22%	Potassium 155mg	* Percent Daily Values are based on a 2,000 calorie diet. Your daily values may be higher or lower, depending on your calorie needs.	
Sodium* 60mg 3%			

Chicken Fryer Leg Quarters

- Leg quarters can be deep-fried, broiled, grilled or roasted.
- To broil or grill, cook the quarters for 40 to 45 minutes or to an internal temperature of 165°F (74°C). Turn once.
- To roast, cook in a preheated 350°F (177°C) oven for 45 to 50 minutes. The quarters are done when juices run clear, 165°F (74°C).

Tip: The drumstick and thigh, leg quarters, can be easily separated at the joint by cutting between the joined two pieces.

Nutrition Facts	Amount Per 3-Ounce (85-Gram) Serving, (cooked)		
Calories 160	Total Carbohydrate* 0g 0%	Vitamin A*	2%
Calories from Fat 60	Dietary Fiber* 0g 0%	Vitamin C*	0%
Total Fat* 7g 11%	Sugars 0g	Calcium*	2%
Saturated Fat* 2g 10%	Protein 23g	Iron*	6%
Cholesterol* 80mg 27%	Potassium 206mg	* Percent Daily Values are based on a 2,000 calorie diet. Your daily values may be higher or lower, depending on your calorie needs.	
Sodium* 75mg 3%			

Whole Turkey

* Roast a whole turkey in a preheated 325°F (163°C) oven for 15 to 18 minutes per pound (.45kg). Add 20 minutes to the total time if the turkey is stuffed. It is done when the temperature at the inner thigh is 180°F (82°C) and the temperature of the stuffing is 165°F (74°C). Let turkey rest 10 minutes before carving. A whole turkey may also be deep-fried, but this requires special equipment.

Tip: Don't over-stuff a turkey; the stuffing expands as it heats.

Nutrition Facts		Amount Per 3-Ounce (85-Gram) Serving, (cooked)			
Calories	140	Total Carbohydrate*	0g	0%	Vitamin A*	0%
Calories from Fat	40	Dietary Fiber*	0g	0%	Vitamin C*	0%
Total Fat*	4g	6%	Sugars	0g	Calcium*	2%
Saturated Fat*	1.5g	8%	Protein	25g	Iron*	8%
Cholesterol*	65mg	22%	Potassium	253mg	* Percent Daily Values are based on a 2,000 calorie diet. Your daily values may be higher or lower, depending on your calorie needs.
Sodium*	60mg	3%			

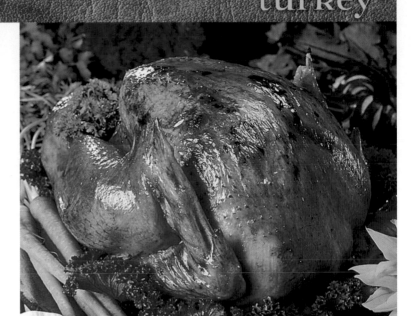

Baked Whole Turkey

Turkey Breast

* Roast whole in a preheated 325°F (163°C) oven for 22 to 25 minutes per pound (.45kg) with bone-in or until the internal temperature reaches 165°F (74°C). Let breast rest 10 minutes before carving. A whole turkey breast may be deep-fried, but this requires special equipment.

Tip: Roasting a turkey breast instead of a whole turkey at Thanksgiving is a smart choice for smaller gatherings, and the leftovers make delicious sandwiches.

Nutrition Facts		Amount Per 3-Ounce (85-Gram) Serving, (cooked)			
Calories	110	Total Carbohydrate*	0g	0%	Vitamin A*	0%
Calories from Fat	5	Dietary Fiber*	0g	0%	Vitamin C*	0%
Total Fat*	1g	1%	Sugars	0g	Calcium*	2%
Saturated Fat*	0g	0%	Protein	26g	Iron*	8%
Cholesterol*	70mg	23%	Potassium	248mg	* Percent Daily Values are based on a 2,000 calorie diet. Your daily values may be higher or lower, depending on your calorie needs.
Sodium*	45mg	2%			

Turkey Drumsticks

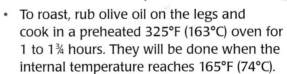

* Turkey drumsticks can be roasted, braised or cooked in a crockpot.
* To roast, rub olive oil on the legs and cook in a preheated 325°F (163°C) oven for 1 to 1¾ hours. They will be done when the internal temperature reaches 165°F (74°C).
* To braise, brown the legs, add 2 cups (473ml) liquid, cover and simmer until meat is so tender it slips off the bone (about 1 to 1½ hours, depending on the size of the legs).

Tip: Don't add salt to chicken stock because the flavors concentrate as the liquid reduces.

Nutrition Facts		Amount Per 3-Ounce (85-Gram) Serving, (cooked)			
Calories	140	Total Carbohydrate*	0g	0%	Vitamin A*	0%
Calories from Fat	45	Dietary Fiber*	0g	0%	Vitamin C*	0%
Total Fat*	4.5g	8%	Sugars	0g	Calcium*	0%
Saturated Fat*	1.5g	8%	Protein	24g	Iron*	10%
Cholesterol*	60mg	20%	Potassium	214mg	* Percent Daily Values are based on a 2,000 calorie diet. Your daily values may be higher or lower, depending on your calorie needs.
Sodium*	70mg	2%			

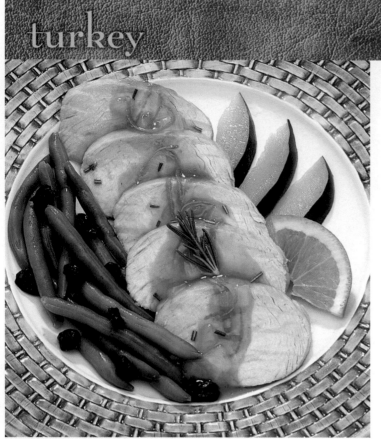

Turkey Breast Roast, Boneless

Turkey Wings

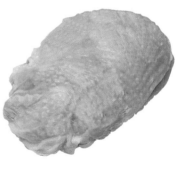

- Brown in a skillet or broiler. Place in a casserole; add ½ to 2 cups (118ml to 473ml) liquid. Cover and cook in a preheated 350°F (177°C) oven for 1 to 1½ hours, or until meat is so tender it slips off the bone.

Tip: Big, meaty turkey wings in Buffalo sauce make an attention-getting mini-meal or appetizer for parties and other casual gatherings.

Nutrition Facts	Amount Per 3-Ounce (85-Gram) Serving, meat & skin, (cooked)			
Calories	190	Total Carbohydrate* 0g 0%	Vitamin A*	0%
Calories from Fat 90		Dietary Fiber* 0g 0%	Vitamin C*	0%
Total Fat*	10g 15%	Sugars 0g	Calcium*	2%
Saturated Fat*	3g 13%	Protein 23g	Iron*	6%
Cholesterol*	70mg 23%	Potassium 230mg	* Percent Daily Values are based on a 2,000 calorie diet. Your daily values may be higher or lower, depending on your calorie needs.	
Sodium*	55mg 2%			

Turkey Thighs

- To barbecue boned thighs, marinate them overnight, then cook over medium-hot coals for 1 to 1¾ hours or until juices run clear or an internal temperature of 180°F (82°C) is reached.

- Thighs are tasty braised. Brown the thighs, add ½ to 2 cups (118 to 473ml) red wine or other liquid and cook at 350°F (177°C) in preheated oven for 1 to 1½ hours. Thighs will be done when the juices run clear or an internal temperature of 165°F (74°C) is reached.

Tip: Stock can be made from the bones of roasted poultry. Cook with liquid, vegetables and herbs.

Nutrition Facts	Amount Per 3-Ounce (85-Gram) Serving, (cooked)			
Calories	130	Total Carbohydrate* 0g 0%	Vitamin A*	0%
Calories from Fat 70		Dietary Fiber* 0g 0%	Vitamin C*	0%
Total Fat*	7g 11%	Sugars 0g	Calcium*	0%
Saturated Fat*	3g 13%	Protein 16g	Iron*	8%
Cholesterol*	55mg 18%	Potassium 205mg	* Percent Daily Values are based on a 2,000 calorie diet. Your daily values may be higher or lower, depending on your calorie needs.	
Sodium*	370mg 15%			

Turkey Breast Roast, Boneless

- Roast in a preheated 325°F (163°C) oven for 15 to 18 minutes per pound (.45kg) or until the internal temperature reaches 165°F (74°C).

Tip: For stuffing, mix butter, onion, bread crumbs, parsley and egg. Roll breast over stuffing and secure with string.

Nutrition Facts	Amount Per 3-Ounce (85-Gram) Serving, (cooked)			
Calories	110	Total Carbohydrate* 0g 0%	Vitamin A*	0%
Calories from Fat 5		Dietary Fiber* 0g 0%	Vitamin C*	0%
Total Fat*	0.5g 1%	Sugars 0g	Calcium*	2%
Saturated Fat*	0g 0%	Protein 26g	Iron*	8%
Cholesterol*	70mg 23%	Potassium 248mg	* Percent Daily Values are based on a 2,000 calorie diet. Your daily values may be higher or lower, depending on your calorie needs.	
Sodium*	45mg 2%			

Turkey Tenderloin

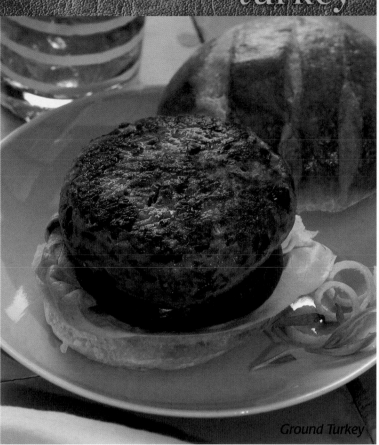

- A versatile cut, these can be grilled, sautéed, divided into cutlets or stir-fried.
- To grill, marinate and then cook over hot coals for 20 minutes. Turn once.
- To roast, cook for 18 to 30 minutes in a preheated oven at 350°F (177°C). Internal temperature should read 165°F (74°C).

Tip: Try coating with Jamaican jerk seasoning before grilling. Remember—the longer you leave the seasoning on before cooking, the more intense (and hot!) the flavor.

Ground Turkey

Nutrition Facts	Amount Per 3-Ounce (85-Gram) Serving, (cooked)			
Calories	130	Total Carbohydrate* 0g 0%	Vitamin A*	0%
Calories from Fat 25		Dietary Fiber* 0g 0%	Vitamin C*	0%
Total Fat*	2.5g 4%	Sugars 0g	Calcium*	2%
Saturated Fat*	1g 5%	Protein 25g	Iron*	6%
Cholesterol*	60mg 20%	Potassium 260mg	* Percent Daily Values are based on a 2,000 calorie diet. Your daily values may be higher or lower, depending on your calorie needs.	
Sodium*	55mg 2%			

Turkey Cutlets

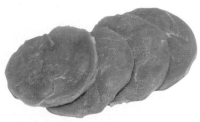

- Sauté ¼-inch-thick (.64cm) turkey cutlets for 3 to 4 minutes per side. Turn once.

Tip: Pound cutlets until thin. Place between layers of wax paper and use a meat mallet until all pieces are the same thickness.

Nutrition Facts	Amount Per 3-Ounce (85-Gram) Serving, (cooked)			
Calories	110	Total Carbohydrate* 0g 0%	Vitamin A*	0%
Calories from Fat 4		Dietary Fiber* 0g 0%	Vitamin C*	0%
Total Fat*	0g 0%	Sugars 0g	Calcium*	0%
Saturated Fat*	0g 0%	Protein 25g	Iron*	8%
Cholesterol*	40mg 13%	Potassium 250mg	* Percent Daily Values are based on a 2,000 calorie diet. Your daily values may be higher or lower, depending on your calorie needs.	
Sodium*	90mg 4%			

Ground Turkey

- Ground turkey is naturally dry because of its low fat content. To make a good burger or meatloaf, add liquid, such as eggs or broth, to the ground turkey. Sauté ¾-inch (1.9cm) patties in 2 tablespoons (30ml) of oil over medium-high heat for 5 to 7 minutes per side. Turn once. Internal temperature should read 165°F (74°C).

Tips: Turkey burgers are a delicious, low-fat alternative to beef. Jazz them up by adding chopped jalapeños and a dash of Worcestershire before making patties.

Nutrition Facts	Amount Per 3-Ounce (85-Gram) Serving, (cooked)			
Calories	200	Total Carbohydrate* 0g 0%	Vitamin A*	0%
Calories from Fat 100		Dietary Fiber* 0g 0%	Vitamin C*	0%
Total Fat*	11g 17%	Sugars 0g	Calcium*	2%
Saturated Fat*	3g 15%	Protein 23g	Iron*	10%
Cholesterol*	85mg 28%	Potassium 230mg	* Percent Daily Values are based on a 2,000 calorie diet. Your daily values may be higher or lower, depending on your calorie needs.	
Sodium*	90mg 4%			

Cornish Game Hen

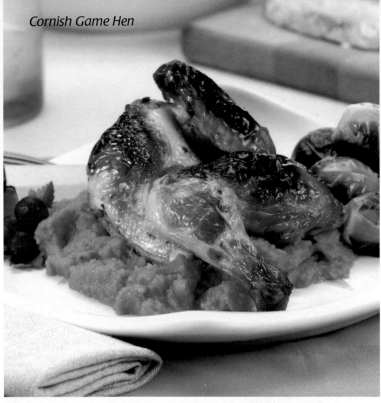

Duck

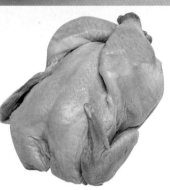

- Roast a whole duck in a preheated oven at 350°F (177°C) for 18 minutes per pound (.45kg).

- For stuffed birds, add 20 minutes to the total roasting time. It will be done when juices run clear or an internal temperature of 180°F (82°C).

- Boneless duck breast may be grilled 8 to 10 minutes over very hot coals or sautéed for 8 to 10 minutes. Turn once.

Tip: Duck pieces may also be braised.

Nutrition Facts	Amount Per 3-Ounce (85-Gram) Serving, meat only, (cooked)				
Calories	170	Total Carbohydrate*	0g	0%	Vitamin A*	2%
Calories from Fat	90	Dietary Fiber*	0g	0%	Vitamin C*	0%
Total Fat*	10g 15%	Sugars	0g		Calcium*	2%
Saturated Fat*	4g 18%	Protein	20g		Iron*	15%
Cholesterol*	75mg 25%	Potassium	214mg		* Percent Daily Values are based on a 2,000 calorie diet. Your daily values may be higher or lower, depending on your calorie needs.	
Sodium*	55mg 2%					

Cornish Game Hens

- Roast in a preheated 350°F (177°C) oven for 1 to 1¼ hours or until the internal temperature of the thigh reads 180°F (82°C).

- Cornish Game Hens can also be split in half and grilled or broiled for 30 minutes.

Tip: Pierce a whole lemon and place in the hen's cavity before baking for a fresh citrus flavor.

Nutrition Facts	Amount Per 3-Ounce (85-Gram) Serving, (cooked)				
Calories	220	Total Carbohydrate*	0g	0%	Vitamin A*	2%
Calories from Fat	140	Dietary Fiber*	0g	0%	Vitamin C*	0%
Total Fat*	15g 23%	Sugars	0g		Calcium*	2%
Saturated Fat*	5g 23%	Protein	19g		Iron*	4%
Cholesterol*	110mg 37%	Potassium	208mg		* Percent Daily Values are based on a 2,000 calorie diet. Your daily values may be higher or lower, depending on your calorie needs.	
Sodium*	55mg 2%					

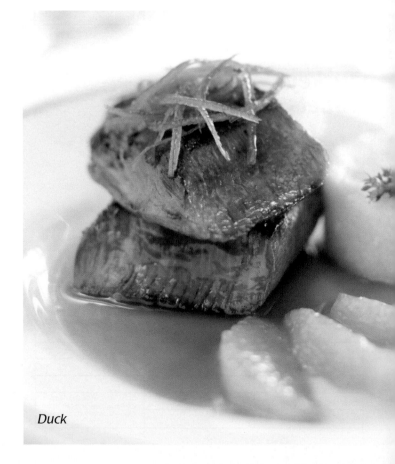

Duck

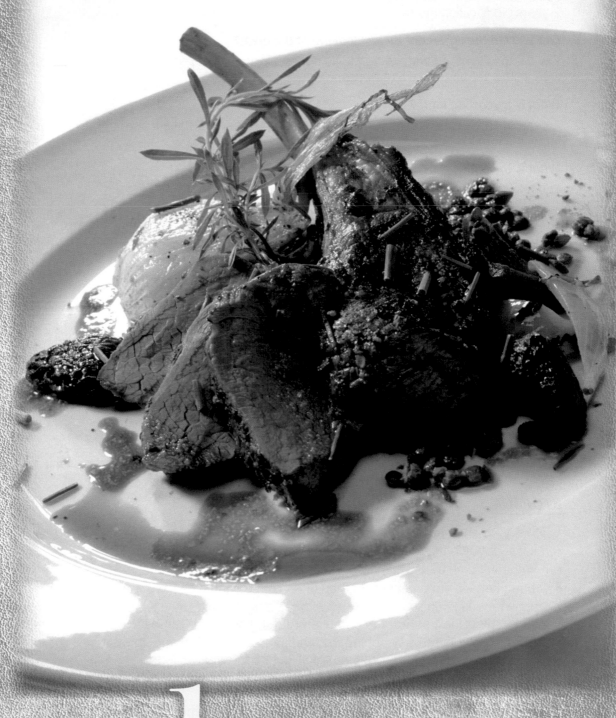

lamb

What's the difference between lamb and mutton?

Lamb comes from sheep that are between 5 months and 1 year old. Meat from sheep more than 2 years old is called mutton.

Can you tell the difference by just looking at the meat?

Yes. Lamb is light red with white fat. Its bones are moist and red. Mutton is dark, almost purplish, with yellow fat and dry white bones.

What is a yearling lamb?

A yearling lamb is between 1 and 2 years old. The meat will have a stronger taste than younger lamb. It should be labeled "yearling lamb."

What is the fell?

The fell is the papery-thin, whitish membrane that coats the lamb.

Why do cookbooks recommend that lamb is best served medium rare?

Lamb loses its delicate taste if it is cooked in a dry heat beyond medium. Many people who don't like lamb have eaten it overcooked.

What is a rack of lamb?

A rack of lamb is similar to the standing rib roast of beef. The rack is, of course, much smaller. A rack of lamb has 7 to 8 ribs but only feeds 2 people.

SELECTION

- Choose lamb that is light red and finely textured. The fat should be white, not yellow. Look for lamb bones that are red and moist.
- Vacuum-packaged lamb from New Zealand or Australia will look purplish until removed from the package.
- Lamb should have a good, fresh smell. Avoid packages with excessive liquid.
- The order of United States Department of Agriculture grading is *Prime, Choice, Good* and *Utility*. Most of what is available in the stores is *Choice*.

STORAGE

- Select your lamb just before checking out at the supermarket.
- If it will not be refrigerated within 30 minutes, place the lamb in a cooler.
- If you don't plan to use the lamb within 2 days, freeze it immediately.
- Ground lamb is more perishable than other cuts. It should be used within 24 hours.
- Store-wrapped lamb should be used within 2 days. Store loosely wrapped (in foil or plastic wrap) lamb in the coldest part of the refrigerator for 4 days. Lamb can be frozen for 6 months.
- Prevent freezer burn by wrapping the lamb in moisture-proof, airtight material, such as food freezer bags or heavy-duty aluminum foil, before freezing.

HANDLING

- Wash hands with hot soapy water for 20 seconds before and after handling lamb.
- Wash knives, counters and cutting boards with hot soapy water immediately after use.
- Do not use the meat knife to cut vegetables without washing the knife and cutting board first.
- Trim as much fat as possible from the lamb.
- Never place cooked lamb back on the same platter used before cooking.
- Always defrost and marinate lamb in the refrigerator, never on the counter.

LAMB CUT	ROAST	GRILL	BROIL	PAN-BROIL	BRAISE
Lamb Breast					X
Lamb Riblets	X	X			X
Lamb Shanks					X
Lamb Stew					X
Lamb Tenderloin				X	
Leg of Lamb	X				
Leg of Lamb, Butterflied		X	X		
Leg Steak		X	X		
Loin Chops		X	X	X	
Loin of Lamb	X	X			
Rack of Lamb	X	X	X		
Rib Chops		X	X	X	
Shoulder Arm Chop		X	X		X
Shoulder Roast					X
Shoulder Roast, Boneless and Rolled	X				X
Sirloin Chop, Boneless		X	X	X	
Sirloin Roast	X	X (Steaks)	X (Steaks)		

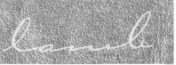

How to pan-broil and braise

- To pan-broil lamb, place lamb in heavy skillet. Do not add fat or water and do not cover. Cook slowly and turn lamb occasionally, pouring off any drippings that accumulate. Cook until lamb is browned on both sides and to desired doneness. Season and serve.

- Braising is a moist heat method of cooking used for both small and large less-tender cuts of lamb. Heat a small amount of fat in a heavy frying pan and brown lamb on all sides. Pour off drippings and season as desired. Add a small amount of liquid such as water, juice, broth or wine. Cover pan tightly and cook at a low temperature until tender.

How to pan-fry

- This dry heat method of cooking is used to cook small, tender cuts of lamb such as loin chops, rib chops, shoulder chops, sirloin steaks, center-cut leg steaks and ground lamb patties. Use this method for thin cuts. Heat a small amount of oil in a heavy frying pan. If the pan smokes, the temperature is too high. Add lamb and brown slowly, turning occasionally.

How to broil and grill

- Because of its natural tenderness, lamb is ideal for outdoor grilling. Boneless rolled roasts should be as cylindrical as possible. Steaks and chops should be at least 1 inch (2.54cm) thick.

- To broil, preheat oven. Place well-trimmed lamb on rack in broiling pan. Brown according to taste and turn halfway through cooking time, to an internal temperature of 145°F (63°C).

- Trim chops, steaks and roasts before cooking to prevent smoke and fire flare-ups. Use tongs when turning to avoid loss of natural juices.

- Place chops, steaks, patties and kabobs on a rack 4 inches (10.16cm) away from coals and cook to desired doneness.

- Chops, steaks and patties must be turned halfway through cooking. Turn kabobs several times and butterflied legs every 10 minutes during cooking.

How to roast

- To roast, preheat oven and place lamb fat side up on rack in open roasting pan. Season as desired. Insert a meat thermometer in the thickest muscle. Take care not to hit a bone or fat. Do not add water. Do not cover. Roast to desired degree of doneness.

- Allow to stand in a warm place for 15 to 20 minutes after removal from the oven to make slicing easier. Cover loosely with a tent of aluminum foil. The roast continues to cook during rest and may gain a few degrees.

Loin of Lamb

- Roast in a 325°F (163°C) preheated oven for 20 minutes per pound (.45kg) for medium rare or until internal temperature reads 145°F (63°C) for medium rare. Let rest for 15 minutes before carving.
- Grill over hot coals for 15 minutes per side for medium rare to an internal temperature of 145°F (63°C). Let rest 15 minutes before carving.

Tip: The simplest seasonings are often the best choice for loin of lamb; rub the cut end of a garlic clove over the meat and then sprinkle well with salt and pepper before cooking.

Nutrition Facts		Amount Per 3-Ounce (85-Gram) Serving, (cooked)			
Calories	170	Total Carbohydrate*	0g 0%	Vitamin A*	0%
Calories from Fat 80		Dietary Fiber*	0g 0%	Vitamin C*	0%
Total Fat*	8g 15%	Sugars	0g	Calcium*	0%
Saturated Fat*	3g 15%	Protein	23g	Iron*	10%
Cholesterol*	75mg 25%	Potassium	227mg	* Percent Daily Values are based on a 2,000 calorie diet. Your daily values may be higher or lower, depending on your calorie needs.	
Sodium*	55mg 2%				

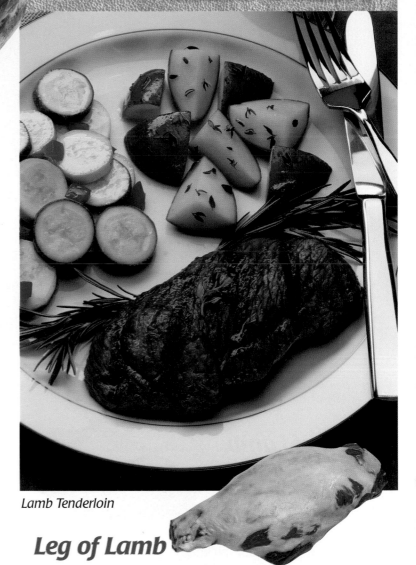

Lamb Tenderloin

Lamb Tenderloin

- Pan-broil in a tablespoon (15ml) of oil in a heavy skillet over medium heat for 8 to 10 minutes. Brown slowly. Turn occasionally. Internal temperature will read 145°F (63°C) for medium rare.

Tip: Lamb is best when kept hot; serve on a warmed platter and provide guests with warm plates.

Leg of Lamb

- Roast a whole leg of lamb in a preheated 350°F (177°C) oven for 20 minutes per pound (.45kg) for medium rare to an internal temperature of 145°F (63°C). Let roast stand 20 minutes.
- A "short leg" shank or sirloin half will cook in about 1¼ hours.

Tip: Leg of lamb is sold boneless, rolled or tied for roasting. A tied leg accommodates stuffing.

Nutrition Facts		Amount Per 3-Ounce (85-Gram) Serving, (cooked)			
Calories	160	Total Carbohydrate*	0g 0%	Vitamin A*	0%
Calories from Fat 70		Dietary Fiber*	0g 0%	Vitamin C*	0%
Total Fat*	7g 11%	Sugars	0g	Calcium*	2%
Saturated Fat*	3g 15%	Protein	23g	Iron*	10%
Cholesterol*	70mg 23%	Potassium	289mg	* Percent Daily Values are based on a 2,000 calorie diet. Your daily values may be higher or lower, depending on your calorie needs.	
Sodium*	70mg 3%				

Nutrition Facts		Amount Per 3-Ounce (85-Gram) Serving, (cooked)			
Calories	210	Total Carbohydrate*	0g 0%	Vitamin A*	0%
Calories from Fat 110		Dietary Fiber*	0g 0%	Vitamin C*	0%
Total Fat*	12g 20%	Sugars	0g	Calcium*	0%
Saturated Fat*	5g 25%	Protein	22g	Iron*	10%
Cholesterol*	80mg 25%	Potassium	271mg	* Percent Daily Values are based on a 2,000 calorie diet. Your daily values may be higher or lower, depending on your calorie needs.	
Sodium*	55mg 2%				

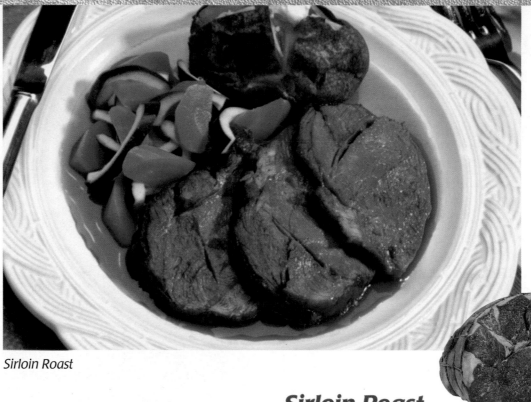

Sirloin Roast

Leg of Lamb, Butterflied

- A butterflied leg of lamb has been de-boned and cut so that it is of equal thickness.
- Grill over moderate coals for about 40 minutes to an internal temperature of 145°F (63°C) for medium rare. Turn once. Let rest for 15 minutes before carving.
- Broil 4 to 5 inches (10.16 to 12.7cm) from the heat source for about 20 minutes per side for rare. Let rest for 15 minutes before carving.

Tip: Marinate butterflied leg in garlic, cumin, oregano, fresh lemon juice and olive oil.

Sirloin Roast, Boneless

- Roast in a preheated 350°F (177°C) oven for 25 minutes per pound (.45kg) to an internal temperature of 145°F (63°C) for medium rare. Let rest for 15 minutes before carving.
- Cut roast into 1-inch (2.54cm) steaks and grill over moderate coals for 10 to 12 minutes for medium rare to an internal temperature of 145°F (63°C). Turn once.
- Broil steaks 4 inches (10.16cm) from the heat source for approximately 10 to 12 minutes or to an internal temperature of 145°F (63°C), for medium rare. Turn once.

Tip: Right before removal from oven, slash the roast in several places and rub in a small amount of butter for added moistness and flavor.

Leg of Lamb, Butterflied — Nutrition Facts

Nutrition Facts Amount Per 3-Ounce (85-Gram) Serving, (cooked)		
Calories 170	Total Carbohydrate* 0g 0%	Vitamin A* 0%
Calories from Fat 70	Dietary Fiber* 0g 0%	Vitamin C* 0%
Total Fat* 8g 12%	Sugars 0g	Calcium* 0%
Saturated Fat* 3g 15%	Protein 24g	Iron* 10%
Cholesterol* 80mg 27%	Potassium 283mg	* Percent Daily Values are based on a 2,000 calorie diet. Your daily values may be higher or lower, depending on your calorie needs.
Sodium* 60mg 3%		

Sirloin Roast, Boneless — Nutrition Facts

Nutrition Facts Amount Per 3-Ounce (85-Gram) Serving, (cooked)		
Calories 240	Total Carbohydrate* 0g 0%	Vitamin A* 0%
Calories from Fat 150	Dietary Fiber* 0g 0%	Vitamin C* 0%
Total Fat* 17g 26%	Sugars 0g	Calcium* 0%
Saturated Fat* 7g 35%	Protein 21g	Iron* 10%
Cholesterol* 80mg 27%	Potassium 258mg	* Percent Daily Values are based on a 2,000 calorie diet. Your daily values may be higher or lower, depending on your calorie needs.
Sodium* 60mg 3%		

Shoulder Roast, Boneless and Rolled

- Preheat oven to 350°F (177°C). Roast for 25 minutes per pound (.45kg) for medium rare to an internal temperature of 145°F (63°C). Let roast rest 15 minutes before carving.

Tip: A meat thermometer is the best guide for checking doneness. Insert into the center of the thickest muscle of the meat. Be careful not to touch fat or bone in bone-in roasts.

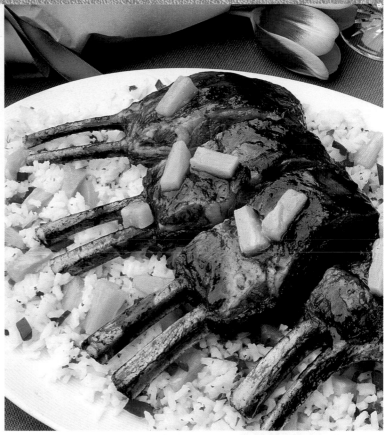

Rack of Lamb

Nutrition Facts		Amount Per 3-Ounce (85-Gram) Serving, (cooked)			
Calories	230	Total Carbohydrate* 0g	0%	Vitamin A*	0%
Calories from Fat 150		Dietary Fiber* 0g	0%	Vitamin C*	0%
Total Fat*	16g 25%	Sugars 0g		Calcium*	2%
Saturated Fat*	7g 35%	Protein 19g		Iron*	10%
Cholesterol*	75mg 25%	Potassium 213mg		* Percent Daily Values are based on a 2,000 calorie diet. Your daily values may be higher or lower, depending on your calorie needs.	
Sodium*	55mg 2%				

Shoulder Roast, Bone-in

- Brown on all sides in a heavy, lidded casserole. Add ½ to 2 cups (188 to 473ml) of liquid. Cover and cook in a preheated 325°F (163°C) oven 25 minutes per pound (.45kg) or until meat is fork-tender.

Tip: Lamb shoulder roast is ideal for stews; consider cutting it into smaller pieces for extra tenderness and reduced cooking time.

Nutrition Facts		Amount Per 3-Ounce (85-Gram) Serving, (cooked)			
Calories	230	Total Carbohydrate* 0g	0%	Vitamin A*	0%
Calories from Fat 140		Dietary Fiber* 0g	0%	Vitamin C*	0%
Total Fat*	16g 25%	Sugars 0g		Calcium*	2%
Saturated Fat*	6g 30%	Protein 20g		Iron*	8%
Cholesterol*	80mg 27%	Potassium 285mg		* Percent Daily Values are based on a 2,000 calorie diet. Your daily values may be higher or lower, depending on your calorie needs.	
Sodium*	70mg 3%				

Rack of Lamb

- To roast, preheat oven to 375°F (191°C). Roast for 30 minutes per pound (.45kg) for medium rare to an internal temperature of 145°F (63°C). Let stand 15 minutes before carving.
- Grill over moderate coals for 25 to 30 minutes for medium rare to an internal temperature of 145°F (63°C).

Tip: A small roast, rack of lamb trimmed and ready for the oven is called frenched. Ideally lamb is cooked until blush pink in the center.

Nutrition Facts		Amount Per 3-Ounce (85-Gram) Serving, (cooked)			
Calories	200	Total Carbohydrate* 0g	0%	Vitamin A*	0%
Calories from Fat 100		Dietary Fiber* 0g	0%	Vitamin C*	0%
Total Fat*	11g 17%	Sugars 0g		Calcium*	2%
Saturated Fat*	4g 20%	Protein 22g		Iron*	8%
Cholesterol*	75mg 25%	Potassium 268mg		* Percent Daily Values are based on a 2,000 calorie diet. Your daily values may be higher or lower, depending on your calorie needs.	
Sodium*	70mg 3%				

lamb

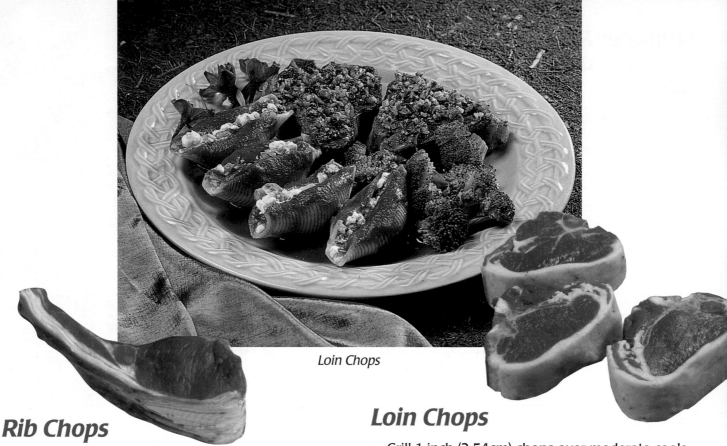

Loin Chops

Rib Chops

- Grill 1-inch (2.54cm) chops over moderate coals for 12 minutes for medium rare to an internal temperature of 145°F (63°C). Turn once.
- Broil 1-inch (2.54cm) chops 3 to 4 inches (7.62 to 10.16cm) from heat source for 12 minutes for medium rare to an internal temperature of 145°F (63°C). Turn once.
- Pan-broil 1-inch (2.54cm) chops over medium high heat in a heavy skillet. Turn when juices appear on top of unseared side. Cook for a total of 8 to 10 minutes for medium rare to an internal temperature of 145°F (63°C). Turn once.

Tip: Rib chops contain more fat and, thus, more flavor than other choices.

Nutrition Facts	Amount Per 3-Ounce (85-Gram) Serving, (cooked)			
Calories	200	Total Carbohydrate* 0g 0%	Vitamin A*	0%
Calories from Fat 110		Dietary Fiber* 0g 0%	Vitamin C*	0%
Total Fat*	11g 15%	Sugars 0g	Calcium*	0%
Saturated Fat*	4g 20%	Protein 22g	Iron*	8%
Cholesterol*	75mg 25%	Potassium 268mg	* Percent Daily Values are based on a 2,000 calorie diet. Your daily values may be higher or lower, depending on your calorie needs.	
Sodium*	70mg 2%			

Loin Chops

- Grill 1-inch (2.54cm) chops over moderate coals for 12 minutes for medium rare to an internal temperature of 145°F (63°C). Turn once.
- Broil 1-inch (2.54cm) chops 3 to 4 inches (7.62 to 10.16cm) from heat source for 12 minutes for medium rare to an internal temperature of 145°F (63°C). Turn once.
- Pan-broil 1-inch (2.54cm) chops over medium high heat in a heavy skillet. Turn when juices appear on top of unseared side. Cook for a total of 8 to 10 minutes for medium rare to an internal temperature of 145°F (63°C). Turn once.

Tip: Grilled lamb chops have a natural sweetness that is deliciously complemented by fruit salsas and chutneys. Top cooked chops with a tablespoon (15ml) or so, and serve more on the side.

Nutrition Facts	Amount Per 3-Ounce (85-Gram) Serving, (cooked)			
Calories	170	Total Carbohydrate* 0g 0%	Vitamin A*	0%
Calories from Fat 80		Dietary Fiber* 0g 0%	Vitamin C*	0%
Total Fat*	8g 15%	Sugars 0g	Calcium*	0%
Saturated Fat*	3g 15%	Protein 23g	Iron*	10%
Cholesterol*	75mg 25%	Potassium 227mg	* Percent Daily Values are based on a 2,000 calorie diet. Your daily values may be higher or lower, depending on your calorie needs.	
Sodium*	55mg 2%			

Shoulder Arm Chops

- Choose shoulder arm chops from near the rib if you want to grill or broil them.
- Grill 1-inch (2.54cm) chops over moderate coals for 12 minutes for medium rare to an internal temperature of 145°F (63°C). Turn once.
- Broil 1-inch (2.54cm) chops 3 to 4 inches (7.62 to 10.16cm) from heat source for 12 minutes for medium rare to an internal temperature of 145°F (63°C). Turn once.
- To braise, brown on each side for 3 minutes. Add liquid, reduce heat and cook until fork-tender, about 45 minutes to 1 hour.

Tip: Try braising in a herb-flavored sauce.

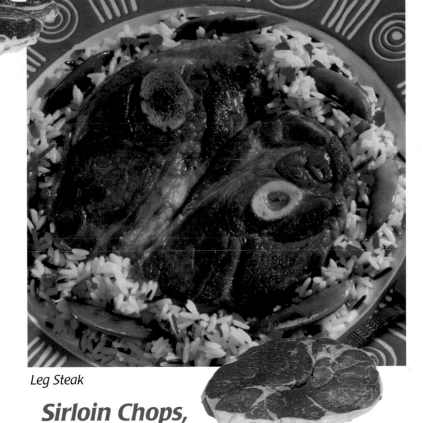

Leg Steak

Nutrition Facts	Amount Per 3-Ounce (85-Gram) Serving, (cooked)			
Calories	230	Total Carbohydrate*	0g 0%	Vitamin A*	0%
Calories from Fat 140		Dietary Fiber*	0g 0%	Vitamin C*	0%
Total Fat*	15g 25%	Sugars	0g	Calcium*	0%
Saturated Fat*	7g 35%	Protein	21g	Iron*	10%
Cholesterol*	80mg 25%	Potassium	267mg	* Percent Daily Values are based on a 2,000 calorie diet. Your daily values may be higher or lower, depending on your calorie needs.
Sodium*	65mg 2%			

Leg Steak

- Grill 1-inch (2.54cm) steaks over moderate coals for 12 minutes for medium rare to an internal temperature of 145°F (63°C). Turn once.
- Broil 1-inch (2.54cm) steaks 3 to 4 inches (7.62 to 10.16cm) from the heat source for 12 minutes for medium rare to an internal temperature of 145°F (63°C). Turn once.

Tip: Lamb's delicate texture can be overwhelmed by acidic marinades made from citrus, vinegar or wine, so don't marinate for more than 16 hours in the refrigerator.

Sirloin Chops, Boneless

- Grill 1-inch (2.54cm) chops over moderate coals for 12 minutes for medium rare to an internal temperature of 145°F (63°C). Turn once.
- Broil 1-inch (2.54cm) chops 3 to 4 inches (7.62 to 10.16cm) from heat source for 12 minutes for medium rare to an internal temperature of 145°F (63°C). Turn once.
- Pan-broil a boneless 1-inch (2.54cm) chop over medium high heat in a heavy, nonstick skillet for 8 to 10 minutes for medium rare to an internal temperature of 145°F (63°C). Turn once.

Tip: Boneless chops are delicious stuffed; cut a deep slit in the side and stuff with your favorite flavor combinations, from chopped apples and sausage to herbed bread crumbs.

Nutrition Facts	Amount Per 3-Ounce (85-Gram) Serving, (cooked)			
Calories	170	Total Carbohydrate*	0g 0%	Vitamin A*	0%
Calories from Fat 70		Dietary Fiber*	0g 0%	Vitamin C*	0%
Total Fat*	8g 12%	Sugars	0g	Calcium*	0%
Saturated Fat*	3g 15%	Protein	24g	Iron*	10%
Cholesterol*	80mg 27%	Potassium	283mg	* Percent Daily Values are based on a 2,000 calorie diet. Your daily values may be higher or lower, depending on your calorie needs.
Sodium*	60mg 3%			

Nutrition Facts	Amount Per 3-Ounce (85-Gram) Serving, (cooked)			
Calories	270	Total Carbohydrate*	0g 0%	Vitamin A*	0%
Calories from Fat 180		Dietary Fiber*	0g 0%	Vitamin C*	0%
Total Fat*	20g 31%	Sugars	0g	Calcium*	2%
Saturated Fat*	8g 40%	Protein	21g	Iron*	8%
Cholesterol*	85mg 28%	Potassium	278mg	* Percent Daily Values are based on a 2,000 calorie diet. Your daily values may be higher or lower, depending on your calorie needs.
Sodium*	65mg 3%			

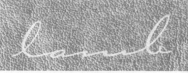

Lamb Stew

- Brown in a heavy, lidded casserole. You may also brown root vegetables such as carrots, potatoes or parsnips. Add enough liquid to cover meat, about 2 cups (473ml). Cover and simmer over low heat until meat is tender, about 1 to 1½ hours.

Tip: For a fragrant flair, add dried fruit such as apricots, prunes, raisins and cranberries.

Nutrition Facts	Amount Per 3-Ounce (85-Gram) Serving, (cooked)			
Calories 180	Total Carbohydrate* 0g	0%	Vitamin A*	0%
Calories from Fat 80	Dietary Fiber* 0g	0%	Vitamin C*	0%
Total Fat* 8g 10%	Sugars 0g		Calcium*	0%
Saturated Fat* 3g 15%	Protein 24g		Iron*	10%
Cholesterol* 80mg 25%	Potassium 292mg		* Percent Daily Values are based on a 2,000 calorie diet. Your daily values may be higher or lower, depending on your calorie needs.	
Sodium* 65mg 2%				

Lamb Riblets

- Moist heat, braising is perfect for riblets. Brown and add liquid. Cover and cook slowly 1 to 2 hours.
- Grill racks of riblets over moderate coals for 15 to 20 minutes.

Tip: Lamb spareribs or riblets can be substituted in your favorite rib recipe with barbecue sauce.

Nutrition Facts	Amount Per 3-Ounce (85-Gram) Serving, (cooked)			
Calories 200	Total Carbohydrate* 0g	0%	Vitamin A*	0%
Calories from Fat 100	Dietary Fiber* 0g	0%	Vitamin C*	0%
Total Fat* 11g 15%	Sugars 0g		Calcium*	0%
Saturated Fat* 4g 20%	Protein 24g		Iron*	10%
Cholesterol* 75mg 25%	Potassium 266mg		* Percent Daily Values are based on a 2,000 calorie diet. Your daily values may be higher or lower, depending on your calorie needs.	
Sodium* 70mg 4%				

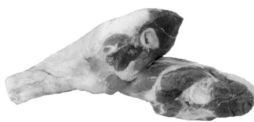

Lamb Shanks

- Brown in a heavy, lidded casserole. Add 2 cups (473ml) of liquid — wine or broth. Cover and place in a preheated 325°F (163°C) oven. Cook for 1½ to 2 hours. Meat should slide off the bone.

Tip: Lamb shanks are ideal braised; add dried fruit, such as figs or raisins, to the cooking liquid for a delicious flavor pairing.

Nutrition Facts	Amount Per 3-Ounce (85-Gram) Serving, (cooked)			
Calories 150	Total Carbohydrate* 0g	0%	Vitamin A*	0%
Calories from Fat 50	Dietary Fiber* 0g	0%	Vitamin C*	0%
Total Fat* 6g 8%	Sugars 0g		Calcium*	0%
Saturated Fat* 2g 10%	Protein 24g		Iron*	10%
Cholesterol* 75mg 25%	Potassium 291mg		* Percent Daily Values are based on a 2,000 calorie diet. Your daily values may be higher or lower, depending on your calorie needs.	
Sodium* 55mg 2%				

Lamb Breast

- Brown, then add 2 cups (473ml) liquid. Cover and simmer on low heat for 1 to 2 hours.
- Another option is to make a pocket between the meat and the ribs of a 1½-pound (.68kg) breast. Stuff with your favorite stuffing. Tie with string at 1-inch (2.54cm) intervals. Roast in a 350°F (177°C) oven until internal temperature reaches 145°F (63°C) for medium rare. Cut between string to make chops.

Tip: Make ahead, refrigerate and remove fat layer before reheating and serving.

Nutrition Facts	Amount Per 3-Ounce (85-Gram) Serving, (cooked)			
Calories 180	Total Carbohydrate* 0g	0%	Vitamin A*	0%
Calories from Fat 70	Dietary Fiber* 0g	0%	Vitamin C*	0%
Total Fat* 8g 12%	Sugars 0g		Calcium*	2%
Saturated Fat* 3g 15%	Protein 24g		Iron*	10%
Cholesterol* 80mg 27%	Potassium 292mg		* Percent Daily Values are based on a 2,000 calorie diet. Your daily values may be higher or lower, depending on your calorie needs.	
Sodium* 65mg 3%				

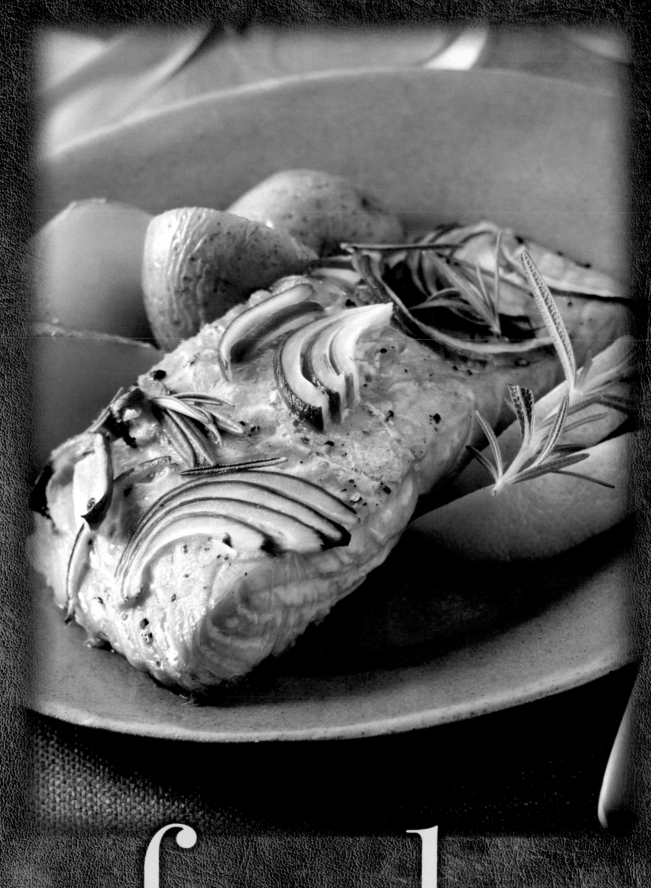

seafood

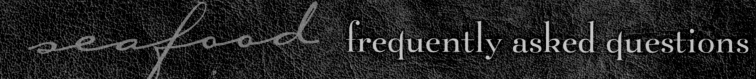

Is there an easy way to determine how long to cook fish?

Yes. Measure the thickest part of the fish and cook 10 minutes for every inch (2.54cm) of thickness. It is often known as the "10-Minute Rule." Be aware that this does not pertain to cooking fish in a microwave.

Can you cook frozen seafood without defrosting it first?

Yes. Just double the time. In other words, cook for 16 to 20 minutes for every inch (2.54cm) of thickness.

How can you tell when fish is done?

Use an instant-read internal thermometer. The USDA recommends 145°F (63°C) for doneness.

Is that the only way?

No, you can trust your eyes. Using a knife in the thickest part of the fish, separate the flesh. Properly done fish should flake easily. The center flesh should be nearly opaque.

How can you tell when mollusks are done?

Clam, mussel and oyster shells will open when they are done. Occasionally, some won't open. Discard them.

Is it safe to eat raw fish?

Millions of people do. However, they do run the risk of bacterial infection. Solid portions of fish must cook to 145°F (63°C), stuffed to 165°F (74°C), to kill bacteria. Elderly people, pregnant women, children and people with chronic illnesses, including liver disease, alcoholic cirrhosis, Diabetes Mellitus, AIDS, compromised immune systems and cancer should NEVER eat raw fish or shellfish.

How can fatty fish be good for you?

So-called fatty fishes are high in omega-3 oils. These oils are beneficial for heart health. Omega-3s reduce the bad cholesterol (LDL) and increase the good cholesterol (HDL).

Which fish have the highest amounts of omega-3 oils?

Best sources of omega-3s are anchovies, sardines, herring, mackerel, bluefish, tuna, salmon, butterfish and pompano. Eel is the only fatty fish with a low level of omega-3 oil.

What is a "dressed fish?"

This is a fish that has been gutted, scaled and had the gills removed. A dressed fish is one that is ready to cook.

What is the difference between steaks and fillets?

Fillets are boneless sections of flesh cut from either side of the fish. Steaks are crosswise cuts of fish that include a small portion of the backbone.

What's the best way to keep mollusks, crabs and lobsters alive once you get them home?

Lobsters should be cooked the day they are purchased. Mollusks can be kept a day or two. Live seafood needs fresh air and moisture. Do not store in closed plastic bags. Keep moist with wet paper towels. If the lobsters don't move when prodded, or the mollusks don't shut when tapped, discard them.

SELECTION

- Fresh fish should have a mild ocean scent. Do not buy if it has an odor.
- Check the "sell by" or "use by" date. Do not buy if it has expired.
- When buying bivalves, such as clams, ask to see the tag that verifies they came from safe waters. (Stores are required to keep these tags for 90 days.)
- When buying whole fish, look for clear, shiny eyes, pink or red gills and tight, shiny scales.
- Don't buy frozen fish if there is evidence of ice crystals or freezer burn.
- Live lobsters and crabs should show movement in their legs.
- Live mollusks may be open, but when tapped, they should close immediately. Discard any that don't.
- Freshly shucked scallops and oysters have a mild sea scent. Oysters will have a slightly milky liquid surrounding them.

SAFE STORAGE

- Purchase seafood right before checking out at the supermarket.
- If seafood will not be refrigerated within 30 minutes, put it in a cooler.
- Seafood should be used within 36 hours of purchase or immediately frozen.
- Defrosted seafood should be used within 36 hours.
- Seafood that is frozen at home (not commercially) should be used within 6 months.

HANDLING

- Always wash hands with hot, soapy water for 20 seconds before and after handling seafood.
- Use separate knives and cutting boards for raw meat and seafood.
- Thaw frozen seafood in the refrigerator, under cold running water. Or, in the microwave oven (according to manufacturer's instructions), if you are going to cook it promptly.
- Allow one day for seafood to defrost in the refrigerator.
- Never defrost seafood on the counter.
- Don't marinate seafood in a citrus-based marinade for more than 30 minutes, or it will begin to "cook."
- Marinade that has been used for seafood must be boiled before it can be used as a sauce after cooking.
- Never put cooked seafood on the same platter used before it was cooked.
- Keep raw seafood separate from cooked seafood to avoid cross-contamination.

The time is right

Fish is a fabulous fast food—it's best cooked quickly over high heat. Just remember the 10-Minute Rule: For every inch (2.54cm) of thickness, bake fish at 450°F (232°C) for 10 minutes. For delicious baked fish:

- Measure fish at the thickest part to estimate cooking time. If ends are thin, fold them under for even cooking.

- If fish is more or less than an inch (2.54cm) thick, add or subtract time from the 10-Minute Rule. For example, if fish is half an inch (1.27cm) thick, divide 10 minutes in half and cook for 5 minutes; if fish is an inch and a half (3.81cm) thick, add 5 minutes and cook for 15 minutes.

- Add an extra 5 minutes if fish is wrapped in foil or covered in sauce.

- Lengthen cooking time if fish is still frozen. Cook to internal temperature of 145°F (63°C) for solid portions of fish, 165°F (74°C) for stuffed fish.

- Do not apply the 10-Minute Rule when using a microwave oven to cook fish.

Keep an eye on it

It's easy to tell when seafood is done by the way it looks. Seafood is done when . . .

> it turns opaque.
>
> it begins to flake easily with a fork (insert fork into the thickest part of the fish to test for doneness).

Broiling and grilling pointers

- Place fish that is 1 inch (2.54cm) thick or less 2 to 4 inches (5.08 to 10.16cm) from the heat source; thicker fish should be placed 5 to 6 inches (12.7 to 15.24cm) away from the broiler.

- Turn fish halfway through cooking time—if fish is under half an inch (1.27cm) thick, don't turn.

- Shellfish cook more quickly than finfish, so cook just until they turn opaque.

- Coat broiling rack with nonstick cooking spray before broiling.

- Baste fish with an oil-based marinade for moistness.

- Baste fish frequently while broiling.

- Thread fish chunks, shrimp or small whole fish on skewers; soak wooden skewers in water for 30 minutes before broiling.

- The easiest way to grill fish is in a grilling basket. The hinged, mesh basket allows you to turn the fish without it breaking apart or sticking.

- Leave skin on fish steaks while grilling.

Baking pointers

- Always fully preheat oven before baking fish.

- Remove fish from the refrigerator at least 20 minutes before baking.

- Prepare whole fish for baking by making several small cuts in the fish.

- Use steaks and fillets of equal size to ensure even cooking.

- Place fillets skin side down.

- Brush fish with melted butter or margarine or oil to keep moist.

- When done, the fish's internal temperature on a cooking thermometer should be 145°F (63°C). Stuffed fish, 165°F (74°C).

- Let baked fish rest 3 to 4 minutes before serving.

Pan-frying pointers

- Clarified butter or margarine works best when pan-frying because it burns less easily.

- If the pan is not preheated, the fish will stick to the pan.

- Drain pan-fried fish by placing it on a paper towel before serving.

- Dredge fillets in seasoned flour, cornmeal or bread crumbs and shake off the excess.

- Use only half the amount of margarine, butter or oil if using a nonstick pan; avoid using aluminum or stainless steel pans.

- Allow margarine, butter or oil to become very hot—but not smoking—before adding fillets.

- Make sure the surface of the fish is thoroughly dry to avoid spatters.

- Give fish plenty of cooking room—don't crowd fillets.

- Sear fish over medium-high heat.

- Turn fish only once halfway through cooking time.

- Fish is ready to turn when the edges start turning crisp and the flesh begins to become opaque.

- Once fish has been seared on both sides, reduce heat to medium until fish is opaque all the way through.

- While pan-frying, keep cooked fish in a warm oven until all of it is done. Do not keep in the oven for more than 20 minutes or fish will become dry.

- Save dry or overcooked fish by serving it with a sauce or by drizzling melted butter over it.

SEAFOOD	BAKE	GRILL	BROIL	PAN-FRY	DEEP-FRY	SAUTÉ	BRAISE	POACH	STEAM	BOIL	RAW*
Catfish	X	X	X	X	X		X				
Clams	X				X				X		X
Cod	X		X	X	X			X	X		
Crab, Dungeness		X	X						X		
Crab, King		X	X						X		
Crab, Snow		X	X						X		
Flounder	X		X	X	X		X	X			
Grouper	X	X	X	X	X		X	X			
Haddock	X	X	X	X	X		X	X	X		
Halibut	X	X	X	X			X	X	X		
Kingfish				X	X		X	X			
Lingcod		X		X							
Lobster, American		X							X	X	
Lobster, Spiny		X	X						X	X	
Mackerel, Atlantic/Pacific		X	X	X							X
Mahi Mahi	X	X	X	X	X	X					
Monkfish			X		X			X	X		
Mussels	X		X						X		X
Octopus		X		X		X		X		X	X
Orange Roughy	X		X	X		X			X		
Oysters	X		X		X				X		X
Perch, Ocean	X		X	X		X					
Pollock	X		X	X	X	X		X	X		
Rockfish	X		X	X		X		X			
Salmon, Atlantic	X	X	X					X			
Scallops, Sea	X	X	X	X	X	X		X			X
Sea Bass	X	X	X	X		X					
Seatrout	X		X	X		X					X
Shark		X		X	X	X					X
Sheepshead	X		X								
Shrimp	X	X	X		X	X			X	X	X
Shrimp, Gulf	X	X	X		X	X			X	X	X
Shrimp, Rock	X	X	X			X			X		
Snapper	X	X	X	X		X		X			
Sole	X			X	X	X		X			
Squid/Calamari						X					X
Swordfish	X	X	X			X		X			
Tuna (White), Albacore		X		X							X
Tuna (Yellowfin)	X	X	X						X	X	X
Tilapia	X	X	X	X		X					
Trout, Rainbow	X	X	X	X	X	X		X	X		

* Elderly people, pregnant women, children, people with chronic illnesses and compromised immune systems should NEVER eat raw fish or shellfish.

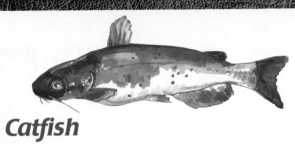

Catfish

Catfish, also known as channel cats, are easily identified by their long whiskers called *barbels*.
Source: Most catfish are farm-raised in Mississippi, Alabama, Arkansas or Louisiana.
Selection and Handling: The flesh of catfish should be white or off-white. Avoid any with red, brown, gray, or yellow coloring. Look for fresh or frozen catfish sold whole or cut into fillets or steaks. Whole fish average 1 to 1½ pounds (454 to 680g) each and fillets average 5 to 15 ounces (142 to 426g) each.
Flavor: Farm-raised catfish taste mild with a slight sweetness due to their controlled diet. Wild catfish may taste slightly "muddy."
Flesh: Firm texture with a slight flakiness.
Preparation: Traditionally coated with cornmeal and fried, catfish also taste great grilled, broiled or baked.

Nutrition Facts	Amount Per 3-Ounce (85-Gram) Serving, (cooked)		
Calories	130	Total Carbohydrate* 0g 0%	Vitamin A* 0%
Calories from Fat 60		Dietary Fiber* 0g 0%	Vitamin C* 0%
Total Fat* 7g 10%		Sugars 0g	Calcium* 0%
Saturated Fat* 1.5g 8%		Protein 16g	Iron* 4%
Cholesterol* 55mg 20%		Potassium 273mg	* Percent Daily Values are based on a 2,000 calorie diet. Your daily values may be higher or lower, depending on your calorie needs.
Sodium* 70mg 2%			

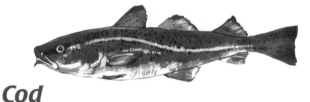

Cod

Cod is one of the most versatile fish. It is eaten fresh, frozen, salted, smoked, pickled, and as breaded fish portions or sticks.
Source: Most cod comes from the northern Atlantic regions of Canada and the United States. The Gulf of Alaska and the Bering Sea have recently become major suppliers.
Selection and Handling: Cod can range from 3 to 245 pounds (1.3 to 111.3kg). The term scrod more accurately refers to smaller cod, those weighing less than 2½ pounds (1.14kg). Avoid fish fillets with separating, as this indicates age. Be sure to cook cod to 145°F (63°C) before eating because parasites are a potential hazard.
Flavor: Very mild.
Flesh: Firm with very large flakes.
Preparation: Cod is especially suited to baking, broiling, steaming and poaching.

Nutrition Facts	Amount Per 3-Ounce (85-Gram) Serving, (cooked)		
Calories	90	Total Carbohydrate* 0g 0%	Vitamin A* 0%
Calories from Fat 5		Dietary Fiber* 0g 0%	Vitamin C* 0%
Total Fat* 0.5g 0%		Sugars 0g	Calcium* 0%
Saturated Fat* 0g 0%		Protein 19g	Iron* 2%
Cholesterol* 45mg 15%		Potassium 207mg	* Percent Daily Values are based on a 2,000 calorie diet. Your daily values may be higher or lower, depending on your calorie needs.
Sodium* 65mg 2%			

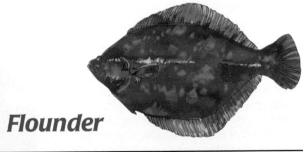

Flounder

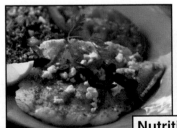

Flounder are part of a large species of flatfish with bodies compressed laterally into flat oval shapes. They are valued for their fine texture and delicate flavor. Some members of the flounder family include dab and plaice. Many fish marketed in North America as fillet of sole are actually flounders.
Source: Gray sole flounder and lemon sole flounder are found in the North Atlantic. Rock sole flounder is found along the Pacific coast. Dab flounder and yellowtail flounder are found along both northern coasts of North America.
Selection and Handling: The size of flounder varies from 4 ounces to 20 pounds (113g to 9kg). They are sold whole, dressed or as fillets.
Flavor: Delicate.
Flesh: Firm and white with a fine texture.
Preparation: Flounder may be cooked by almost any method. Whole flounder are often stuffed.

Nutrition Facts	Amount Per 3-Ounce (85-Gram) Serving, (cooked)		
Calories	100	Total Carbohydrate* 0g 0%	Vitamin A* 0%
Calories from Fat 10		Dietary Fiber* 0g 0%	Vitamin C* 0%
Total Fat* 1.5g 0%		Sugars 0g	Calcium* 0%
Saturated Fat* 0g 0%		Protein 21g	Iron* 0%
Cholesterol* 60mg 20%		Potassium 292mg	* Percent Daily Values are based on a 2,000 calorie diet. Your daily values may be higher or lower, depending on your calorie needs.
Sodium* 90mg 4%			

Grouper are members of the sea bass family. They are also called sand perch, rock cod, coney and jewfish. The most commonly available are black and red groupers.

Source: Grouper come from the Gulf of Mexico, north and south Atlantic Ocean, Pacific Ocean and the Caribbean.

Selection and Handling: Most market fish range from 5 to 10 pounds (2.3 to 4.5kg). Avoid fish larger than 10 pounds (4.5kg). Grouper are ideal for filleting. They can be a source of ciguartera poisoning, caused by a toxin from tropical reefs, so know where the fish was harvested.

Flavor: Mild and sweet.

Flesh: Firm with very large flakes.

Preparation: Grouper can be cut into kabob cubes or used in soups. It is excellent baked, poached, steamed, broiled, grilled or battered and deep-fried. The skin should be removed before cooking.

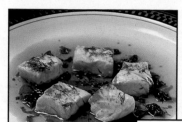

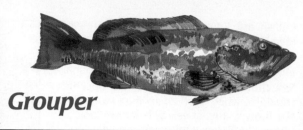

Grouper

Nutrition Facts		Amount Per 3-Ounce (85-Gram) Serving, (cooked)				
Calories	100	Total Carbohydrate*	0g	0%	Vitamin A*	2%
Calories from Fat	10	Dietary Fiber*	0g	0%	Vitamin C*	0%
Total Fat*	1g	0%	Sugars	0g	Calcium*	0%
Saturated Fat*	0g	0%	Protein	21g	Iron*	6%
Cholesterol*	40mg	15%	Potassium	404mg	* Percent Daily Values are based on a 2,000 calorie diet. Your daily values may be higher or lower, depending on your calorie needs.	
Sodium*	45mg	0%				

A member of the cod family, haddock are distinguished from their cousins by a dark lateral line along their sides and a dark spot on their shoulders known, oddly, as both "the devil's thumbprint" and "St. Peter's mark." Haddock are smaller than cod.

Source: Haddock are harvested year-round in the North Atlantic from Newfoundland south to New England and also in the waters off northern Europe.

Selection and Handling: In North America whole haddock are commonly sold fresh. Fresh or frozen fillets and steaks are always sold skin-on to retain their identity.

Flavor: Delicate and mild.

Flesh: White, somewhat finer than cod. Firm texture.

Preparation: Haddock may be prepared by baking, poaching, sautéing and grilling. Because of its mild flavor, haddock should be seasoned lightly.

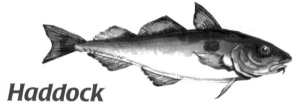

Haddock

Nutrition Facts		Amount Per 3-Ounce (85-Gram) Serving, (cooked)				
Calories	100	Total Carbohydrate*	0g	0%	Vitamin A*	0%
Calories from Fat	5	Dietary Fiber*	0g	0%	Vitamin C*	0%
Total Fat*	1g	0%	Sugars	0g	Calcium*	4%
Saturated Fat*	0g	0%	Protein	21g	Iron*	6%
Cholesterol*	65mg	20%	Potassium	339mg	* Percent Daily Values are based on a 2,000 calorie diet. Your daily values may be higher or lower, depending on your calorie needs.	
Sodium*	75mg	4%				

Halibut is the largest of the flatfish, sometimes attaining weights of 500 pounds (227kg), although more common market weights range between 50 and 100 pounds (23 and 45kg).

Source: Halibut live near the bottom of the ocean. They are harvested along the northern coastlines of both the Atlantic and Pacific oceans. Available year-round, the greatest supply is from March to September.

Selection and Handling: Pacific halibut are often cut into fletches—quartered sections with no bones weighing up to 10 pounds (4.5kg) each. Fresh or frozen halibut steaks and fillets are also available.

Flavor: Mild and sweet.

Flesh: Dense and tender with a firm flake and a crab-like texture.

Preparation: Halibut is best when cooked with moist heat such as poaching, braising or steaming. It may also be grilled, broiled, roasted or sautéed.

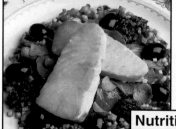

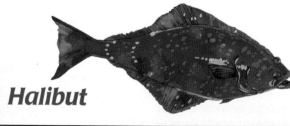

Halibut

Nutrition Facts		Amount Per 3-Ounce (85-Gram) Serving, (cooked)				
Calories	120	Total Carbohydrate*	0g	0%	Vitamin A*	4%
Calories from Fat	25	Dietary Fiber*	0g	0%	Vitamin C*	0%
Total Fat*	2.5g	4%	Sugars	0g	Calcium*	6%
Saturated Fat*	0g	0%	Protein	23g	Iron*	6%
Cholesterol*	35mg	10%	Potassium	490mg	* Percent Daily Values are based on a 2,000 calorie diet. Your daily values may be higher or lower, depending on your calorie needs.	
Sodium*	60mg	2%				

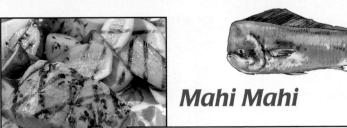

Mahi mahi is also known as dorado, dolphin and dolphin-fish, yet it is not a relative to the marine mammal.

Source: Mahi mahi is found in most of the world's warm waters. It is caught in the Caribbean, off the shores of Florida, near Hawaii and from southern California to Panama.

Selection and Handling: Market size ranges from a few pounds/kilograms to more than 50 pounds (23kg). It is typically sold fresh or frozen as steaks or fillets. Look for consistently colored pink to light beige flesh. It begins to darken and get streaky as it ages.

Flavor: Mild and slightly sweet.

Flesh: Firm with large flakes.

Preparation: For the mildest flavor, remove the tough skin and cut away the dark lateral line before cooking. It may be prepared by any cookery method, but lends itself well to grilling and broiling.

Mahi Mahi

Nutrition Facts		Amount Per 3-Ounce (85-Gram) Serving, (cooked)			
Calories	90	Total Carbohydrate*	0g 0%	Vitamin A*	4%
Calories from Fat	5	Dietary Fiber*	0g 0%	Vitamin C*	0%
Total Fat*	1g 0%	Sugars	0g	Calcium*	0%
Saturated Fat*	0g 0%	Protein	20g	Iron*	6%
Cholesterol*	80mg 25%	Potassium	453mg	* Percent Daily Values are based on a 2,000 calorie diet. Your daily values may be higher or lower, depending on your calorie needs.	
Sodium*	95mg 4%				

Monkfish are also known as goosefish, anglefish, bellyfish, fishing frog and lawyerfish.

Source: In the United States, monkfish are harvested from the Grand Banks to North Carolina.

Selection and Handling: Fishermen trim monkfish on board, saving only the liver (for export to Japan) and the tail for market. They are sold fresh, frozen or as skinless tails and fillets.

Flavor: Very sweet and is nicknamed "poor man's lobster."

Flesh: Extremely firm and white.

Preparation: The tail of the monkfish may be poached or steamed; it is often butterflied and broiled as well. Slices are excellent fried.

Monkfish

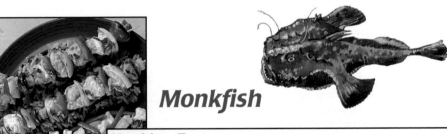

Nutrition Facts		Amount Per 3-Ounce (85-Gram) Serving, (cooked)			
Calories	80	Total Carbohydrate*	0g 0%	Vitamin A*	0%
Calories from Fat	15	Dietary Fiber*	0g 0%	Vitamin C*	0%
Total Fat*	1.5g 2%	Sugars	0g	Calcium*	0%
Saturated Fat*	0g 0%	Protein	16g	Iron*	0%
Cholesterol*	25mg 10%	Potassium	436mg	* Percent Daily Values are based on a 2,000 calorie diet. Your daily values may be higher or lower, depending on your calorie needs.	
Sodium*	20mg 0%				

Orange roughy have reddish bodies and bluish-tinged bellies that turn bright coral after harvest. They average 3 to 4 pounds (1.4 to 1.8kg) each and about 12 inches (30cm) long.

Source: They come from the Tasman Sea in the South Pacific and off the coasts of New Zealand, Australia and Chile. They are caught in very deep waters by huge trawl nets.

Selection and Handling: Orange roughy are most commonly available as fillets. They are usually frozen at sea, thawed on land, cut into fillets and refrozen. Despite the fact it is frozen twice before it gets to retail markets, it holds up extremely well.

Flavor: Delicate, shellfish-like.

Flesh: Tender, firm and dense.

Preparation: Orange roughy are especially suitable for baking, broiling and sautéeing. Any recipe for flounder or sole may be successfully adapted for orange roughy.

Orange Roughy

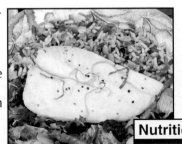

Nutrition Facts		Amount Per 3-Ounce (85-Gram) Serving, (cooked)			
Calories	80	Total Carbohydrate*	0g 0%	Vitamin A*	0%
Calories from Fat	5	Dietary Fiber*	0g 0%	Vitamin C*	0%
Total Fat*	1g 0%	Sugars	0g	Calcium*	4%
Saturated Fat*	0g 0%	Protein	16g	Iron*	0%
Cholesterol*	20mg 8%	Potassium	327mg	* Percent Daily Values are based on a 2,000 calorie diet. Your daily values may be higher or lower, depending on your calorie needs.	
Sodium*	70mg 2%				

Members of the rockfish family, ocean perch are also called redfish, rosefish, red perch and deep-sea perch. Most are a brilliant red to orange color, although some from the Pacific Ocean may be black or yellow.

Source: Pacific Ocean perch inhabit the waters from Alaska to Mexico. Atlantic Ocean perch are found in the continental shelf area, primarily off Canada's and the New England state's coastlines.

Selection and Handling: Ocean perch is marketed fresh or frozen as fillets, but is also available whole. Pacific Ocean perch (sometimes called POP) is usually sold with the skin removed. Atlantic Ocean perch is usually sold with the skin on.

Flavor: Pacific Ocean perch have a delicate flavor. Atlantic Ocean perch have a slightly more distinctive flavor.

Flesh: Medium-firm with a large flake.

Preparation: Ocean perch are excellent baked, broiled or oven-fried.

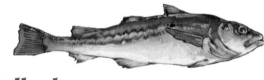

Perch, Ocean

Nutrition Facts			Amount Per 3-Ounce (85-Gram) Serving, (cooked)		
Calories	100		Total Carbohydrate*	0g	0%	Vitamin A*		0%
Calories from Fat	15		Dietary Fiber*	0g	0%	Vitamin C*		0%
Total Fat*	2g	2%	Sugars	0g		Calcium*		10%
Saturated Fat*	0g	0%	Protein	20g		Iron*		6%
Cholesterol*	45mg	15%	Potassium	298mg		* Percent Daily Values are based on a 2,000 calorie diet. Your daily values may be higher or lower, depending on your calorie needs.
Sodium*	80mg	4%				

There are two distinct species of pollock harvested in North America—Atlantic pollock and Pacific pollock—and they differ enormously in taste and texture.

Source: Most Pacific pollock are harvested in the Bering Sea. Atlantic pollock are found on both sides of the northern Atlantic Ocean.

Selection and Handling: Pacific pollock are relatively small and are usually sold as fillets or processed into *surimi* (see page 76). Atlantic pollock are often larger and sold as fillets.

Flavor: Pacific pollock is mild, similar to cod. Atlantic pollock is more distinctively flavored.

Flesh: Pacific is very white and soft with medium flakes. Atlantic is tannish-gray to pink uncooked, while cooked is white with large flakes.

Preparation: Pollock may be prepared by almost any cooking method, but is especially suitable for salads and chowders. Atlantic pollock may be combined with very flavorful herbs and spices.

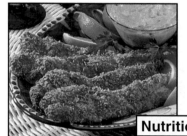

Pollock

Nutrition Facts			Amount Per 3-Ounce (85-Gram) Serving, (cooked)		
Calories	100		Total Carbohydrate*	0g	0%	Vitamin A*		0%
Calories from Fat	10		Dietary Fiber*	0g	0%	Vitamin C*		0%
Total Fat*	1g	0%	Sugars	0g		Calcium*		0%
Saturated Fat*	0g	0%	Protein	20g		Iron*		0%
Cholesterol*	80mg	25%	Potassium	329mg		* Percent Daily Values are based on a 2,000 calorie diet. Your daily values may be higher or lower, depending on your calorie needs.
Sodium*	100mg	4%				

Rockfish are the yelloweye, bocaccio, widow, yellowtail rockfish and ocean perch. The colorful fish have armored gill covers, large heads and spiny fins. They may weigh up to 15 pounds (6.8kg), but average market size is from 1½ to 5 pounds (680g to 2.27kg).

Source: Rockfish are caught from southern California up to British Columbia and Alaska.

Selection and Handling: Rockfish are marketed most commonly as fresh or frozen fillets. Some are sold whole or dressed.

Flavor: Mild, with subtle distinctions among the species. Yelloweye rockfish is considered the best tasting, similar to red snapper.

Flesh: Most are flaky and white. Widow rockfish have a soft flesh that tends to turn brown quickly.

Preparation: Rockfish lend themselves well to any sort of fish cookery method. The yelloweye is best baked or broiled. Others are excellent in soups and chowders, fish cakes and casseroles.

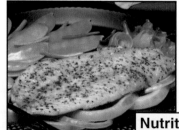

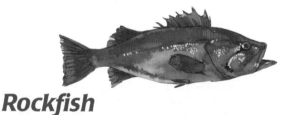

Rockfish

Nutrition Facts			Amount Per 3-Ounce (85-Gram) Serving, (cooked)		
Calories	100		Total Carbohydrate*	0g	0%	Vitamin A*		4%
Calories from Fat	15		Dietary Fiber*	0g	0%	Vitamin C*		0%
Total Fat*	1.5g	2%	Sugars	0g		Calcium*		0%
Saturated Fat*	0g	2%	Protein	20g		Iron*		2%
Cholesterol*	35mg	10%	Potassium	442mg		* Percent Daily Values are based on a 2,000 calorie diet. Your daily values may be higher or lower, depending on your calorie needs.
Sodium*	65mg	2%				

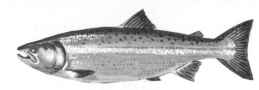

Salmon, Atlantic

Atlantic salmon is predominantly a farmed fish. It is a silver-skinned fish with distinct black cross-like spots over the body and head.

Source: Atlantic salmon is farm-raised in a dozen countries including the United States, United Kingdom, Chile, Norway, Canada, Ireland and Iceland. Countries that farm Atlantic salmon typically add their name to the label. Wild salmon is caught commercially from May to October.

Selection and Handling: Atlantic salmon are sold whole and dressed; as roasts; fillet portions, with skin on or off; and steaks. It is also available as patties, hams and kabobs. Farmed salmon are available year-round.

Flavor: Mild and more delicate than wild salmon.

Flesh: Moderately firm with moist, large flakes.

Preparation: Steaks, fillets and whole fish may be baked, broiled, poached or grilled. Avoid accompanying flavors that may overpower it.

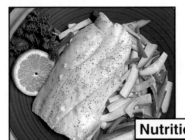

Nutrition Facts		Amount Per 3-Ounce (85-Gram) Serving, (cooked)			
Calories	180	Total Carbohydrate*	0g 0%	Vitamin A*	0%
Calories from Fat	90	Dietary Fiber*	0g 0%	Vitamin C*	6%
Total Fat*	10g 15%	Sugars	0g	Calcium*	0%
Saturated Fat*	2g 10%	Protein	19g	Iron*	0%
Cholesterol*	55mg 20%	Potassium	326mg	* Percent Daily Values are based on a 2,000 calorie diet. Your daily values may be higher or lower, depending on your calorie needs.	
Sodium*	50mg 2%				

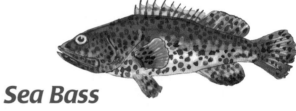

Sea Bass

Sea bass, also known as black sea bass, rock bass or blackfish, have small, stout bodies with smoky gray, brown, or bluish-black skin.

Source: Sea bass occur along the entire Atlantic coast of North America and into the Gulf of Mexico. They're most often found on rocky bottoms near pilings, wrecks and jetties.

Selection and Handling: Black sea bass tend to be about 10 inches (25.4cm) long and range from 1½ to 3¼ pounds (680g to 1.5kg). Usually they're sold whole but may also be found as fillets. If the fish is bought whole, its spiny, spiky dorsal fin should be carefully removed to avoid injury.

Flavor: Very delicate, because of feeding on shrimp and crabs.

Flesh: Firm with very white flesh.

Preparation: Sea bass can be prepared in a variety of ways including frying, baking, broiling, grilling, steaming or sautéing.

Nutrition Facts		Amount Per 3-Ounce (85-Gram) Serving, (cooked)			
Calories	110	Total Carbohydrate*	0g 0%	Vitamin A*	4%
Calories from Fat	20	Dietary Fiber*	0g 0%	Vitamin C*	0%
Total Fat*	2g 3%	Sugars	0g	Calcium*	2%
Saturated Fat*	0.5g 3%	Protein	20g	Iron*	2%
Cholesterol*	45mg 15%	Potassium	279mg	* Percent Daily Values are based on a 2,000 calorie diet. Your daily values may be higher or lower, depending on your calorie needs.	
Sodium*	75mg 3%				

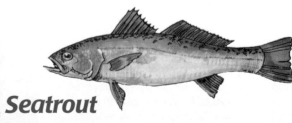

Seatrout

Seatrout are also known as weakfish, referring to the soft tissue around their mouths that tears easily when hooked. This makes fish difficult to land and is considered a challenge for sport fishermen. Seatrout are silvery with small speckles.

Source: Seatrout are found in the Atlantic and part of the Pacific oceans along the coastlines of both North and South America. Harvested by trawlers, gill nets and seines, seatrout have the greatest availability from April to November.

Selection and Handling: Seatrout are available fresh as whole fish, dressed fish or as fillets. Occasionally they're frozen.

Flavor: Sweet and very delicate.

Flesh: White and finely textured.

Preparation: Seatrout is suitable for baking, broiling, grilling and pan-frying. To keep the flesh intact, handle gently and as little as possible.

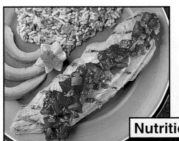

Nutrition Facts		Amount Per 3-Ounce (85-Gram) Serving, (cooked)			
Calories	110	Total Carbohydrate*	0g 0%	Vitamin A*	0%
Calories from Fat	35	Dietary Fiber*	0g 0%	Vitamin C*	0%
Total Fat*	4g 6%	Sugars	0g	Calcium*	0%
Saturated Fat*	1g 6%	Protein	18g	Iron*	0%
Cholesterol*	90mg 30%	Potassium	371mg	* Percent Daily Values are based on a 2,000 calorie diet. Your daily values may be higher or lower, depending on your calorie needs.	
Sodium*	65mg 2%				

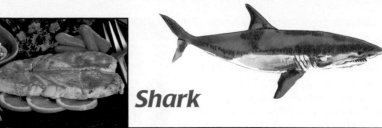

Shark

Sharks are one of the oldest creatures on earth and have changed little in over 33 million years. Although other cultures have eaten shark for centuries, only recently have North Americans begun to appreciate it.

Source: Sharks inhabit all the oceans of the world. The most common shark in North America is the mako, (also known as bonito) which is harvested along the Atlantic coast. Other species are blacktip and dogfish.

Selection and Handling: Shark is typically available fresh or frozen as steaks and fillets.

Flavor: Mild, ranging from bland to slightly sweet. Mako is often compared to swordfish.

Flesh: Very firm, dense and moist. The flesh may be white to pink with red tinges.

Preparation: Trim any dark lines before cooking. Shark is good broiled, grilled, baked and stir-fried well. Marinades and spicy rubs enhance the flavor.

Nutrition Facts		Amount Per 3-Ounce (85-Gram) Serving, (cooked)			
Calories	190	Total Carbohydrate* 5g	0%	Vitamin A*	4%
Calories from Fat 110		Dietary Fiber* 0g	0%	Vitamin C*	0%
Total Fat*	12g 20%	Sugars 0g		Calcium*	4%
Saturated Fat*	2.5g 15%	Protein 16g		Iron*	6%
Cholesterol*	50mg 15%	Potassium 132mg		* Percent Daily Values are based on a 2,000 calorie diet. Your daily values may be higher or lower, depending on your calorie needs.	
Sodium*	105mg 4%				

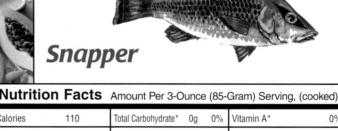

Snapper

Of the over 200 species of snapper, the most common are red, yellowtail, mutton, gray or mangrove, lane and cubera snappers. Only one species may legally be called red snapper.

Source: Snapper are found from North Carolina to Brazil. Most catches are by long-line fishermen in the Gulf of Mexico.

Selection and Handling: Snapper are available year around. Smaller snappers are sold whole or dressed, while larger snappers are often cut into steaks or fillets. All are sold fresh or frozen. Skin color is the key to identifying the species, so the skin is often left on the fish.

Flavor: Mild but distinctive.

Flesh: Moderately firm with a fine flake.

Preparation: Snapper cook well with any technique, but they are especially suited to baking and broiling. The flavor is enhanced by the addition of delicate flavors such as dill weed or lime juice.

Nutrition Facts		Amount Per 3-Ounce (85-Gram) Serving, (cooked)			
Calories	110	Total Carbohydrate* 0g	0%	Vitamin A*	0%
Calories from Fat 15		Dietary Fiber* 0g	0%	Vitamin C*	2%
Total Fat*	1.5g 2%	Sugars 0g		Calcium*	4%
Saturated Fat*	0g 0%	Protein 22g		Iron*	0%
Cholesterol*	40mg 15%	Potassium 444mg		* Percent Daily Values are based on a 2,000 calorie diet. Your daily values may be higher or lower, depending on your calorie needs.	
Sodium*	50mg 2%				

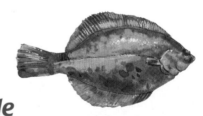

Sole

There are no true soles harvested from the coastal waters of North America. Those marketed as sole are usually flounders (see page 65). True sole is found in European waters and called channel sole or Dover sole. Dover sole ranges from light gray to dark brown with a pale belly. Other varieties of true sole include thickback and sand sole.

Source: Coastal waters from Denmark to the Mediterranean Sea.

Selection and Handling: European Dover sole is usually exported fresh, both whole and dressed. The average size for a whole fish is about 1 pound (454g).

Flavor: Dover sole is light and delicate. Thickback or sand soles are less flavorful than Dover.

Flesh: Firm and white with fine texture.

Preparation: Sole is suited to a variety of cookery methods and flavors. It is excellent fried, baked, broiled, grilled and stuffed.

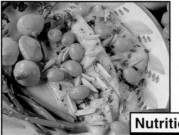

Nutrition Facts		Amount Per 3-Ounce (85-Gram) Serving, (cooked)			
Calories	100	Total Carbohydrate* 0g	0%	Vitamin A*	0%
Calories from Fat 10		Dietary Fiber* 0g	0%	Vitamin C*	0%
Total Fat*	1.5g 0%	Sugars 0g		Calcium*	0%
Saturated Fat*	0g 0%	Protein 21g		Iron*	0%
Cholesterol*	60mg 20%	Potassium 292mg		* Percent Daily Values are based on a 2,000 calorie diet. Your daily values may be higher or lower, depending on your calorie needs.	
Sodium*	90mg 4%				

Swordfish are aptly named for the flat sword-like protrusion that extends from the upper jaw. The "sword" itself may be one-third the length of the body of the fish.

Source: On the Atlantic coast, swordfish is found from Newfoundland to Argentina. On the Pacific coast it's found from California to Chile. It is available year-round, but is most abundant in late spring.

Selection and Handling: Sold as fresh or frozen steaks at least an inch (2.54cm) thick, the flesh may be light gray, orange or pink, depending on the diet of the fish. It should always be highly translucent with a bright sheen.

Flavor: Fairly rich and sweet.

Flesh: Firm (similar to mako shark) and dense.

Preparation: While swordfish may be cooked by any method, it is usually preferred broiled or grilled. Swordfish lends itself to use with flavorful ingredients.

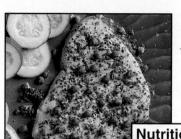

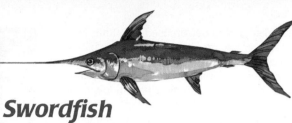

Swordfish

Nutrition Facts		Amount Per 3-Ounce (85-Gram) Serving, (cooked)			
Calories	130	Total Carbohydrate*	0g	0%	Vitamin A*	2%
Calories from Fat	40	Dietary Fiber*	0g	0%	Vitamin C*	0%
Total Fat*	4.5g	6%	Sugars	0g	Calcium*	0%
Saturated Fat*	1g	6%	Protein	22g	Iron*	4%
Cholesterol*	45mg	15%	Potassium	314mg	* Percent Daily Values are based on a 2,000 calorie diet. Your daily values may be higher or lower, depending on your calorie needs.
Sodium*	100mg	4%			

Tombo albacore, also called longfin tuna, are distinguished by long pectoral fins. They generally weigh about 40 pounds (18kg).

Source: Most are caught in the Pacific Ocean, while some are found in the Atlantic Ocean.

Selection and Handling: Select fish that are moist and shiny, avoiding fish that have a rainbow-like sheen or browning on the surface. They are generally sold in steaks, and are best used within a day of purchase.

Flavor: This tuna has a mild flavor.

Flesh: Firm and moist.

Preparation: Tombo albacore are sold without the tough skin. Cut away the dark, reddish flesh and discard. Pan-fry, grill or serve tombo albacore raw as *sashimi*.

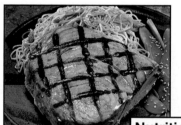

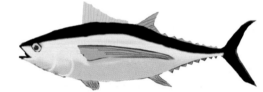

Tuna (White), Albacore

Nutrition Facts		Amount Per 3-Ounce (85-Gram) Serving, (cooked, canned, drained)			
Calories	110	Total Carbohydrate*	0g	0%	Vitamin A*	0%
Calories from Fat	25	Dietary Fiber*	0g	0%	Vitamin C*	0%
Total Fat*	2.5g	4%	Sugars	0g	Calcium*	2%
Saturated Fat*	0.5g	3%	Protein	20g	Iron*	4%
Cholesterol*	35mg	12%	Potassium	200mg	* Percent Daily Values are based on a 2,000 calorie diet. Your daily values may be higher or lower, depending on your calorie needs.
Sodium*	45mg	2%			

Several species of tuna are sold, including yellowfin, bluefin, bigeye, tunny, bonito, ahi and albacore. Usually tuna have elongated silver bodies with bluish backs and large round eyes.

Source: Found mainly in tropical waters. On the eastern shores of North America, yellowfin, bigeye and bluefin are harvested by longline.

Selection and Handling: Select tuna that is deep pink or red (not gray). Avoid any with dry or brown spots or those with flesh that reflects rainbows. Steaks that are at least 1¼ inches (3cm) thick are less likely to dry out during cooking. Use within a day or two of purchase.

Flavor: Delicate but very distinctive.

Flesh: Very firm with a fairly fine flake. Ranges from pink to very deep red in color.

Preparation: Tuna is at its best grilled and is excellent poached or steamed. Because tuna dries out easily, avoid overcooking.

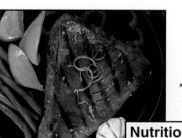

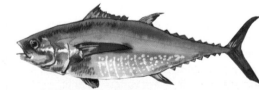

Tuna (Yellowfin)

Nutrition Facts		Amount Per 3-Ounce (85-Gram) Serving, (cooked)			
Calories	120	Total Carbohydrate*	0g	0%	Vitamin A*	2%
Calories from Fat	10	Dietary Fiber*	0g	0%	Vitamin C*	2%
Total Fat*	1g	2%	Sugars	0g	Calcium*	2%
Saturated Fat*	0g	0%	Protein	25g	Iron*	4%
Cholesterol*	50mg	17%	Potassium	485mg	* Percent Daily Values are based on a 2,000 calorie diet. Your daily values may be higher or lower, depending on your calorie needs.
Sodium*	40mg	2%			

Kingfish, not to be confused with King Mackerel, are members of the drum and croaker family. They are a lean fish that rarely grow to more than a foot long. Silver-skinned with soft, white flesh, they have a low omega-3 oil level.

Source: There are 2 varieties of kingfish: northern and southern. Northern kingfish are found in the Atlantic from Maine to Florida. The southern variety is found in the Gulf of Mexico.

Selection and Handling: If the gills are bright red, the kingfish is fresh. If the head has been removed, check the edges of the flesh. There should be no browning.

Flavor: Delicious, sweet and mild.

Flesh: Soft and white.

Preparation: Never serve kingfish raw. Kingfish is good for pan-frying, braising, poaching or deep-frying.

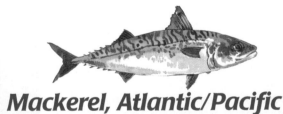

Kingfish

Nutrition Facts		Amount Per 3-Ounce (85-Gram) Serving, (cooked)				
Calories	130	Total Carbohydrate*	0g	0%	Vitamin A*	4%
Calories from Fat	50	Dietary Fiber*	0g	0%	Vitamin C*	0%
Total Fat*	5g	8%	Sugars	0g	Calcium*	6%
Saturated Fat*	1g	6%	Protein	19g	Iron*	6%
Cholesterol*	70mg	25%	Potassium	300mg	* Percent Daily Values are based on a 2,000 calorie diet. Your daily values may be higher or lower, depending on your calorie needs.	
Sodium*	80mg	4%				

Lingcod are not a member of the cod family. Lingcod belong to the greenling family, a group of fish known for their big mouths, lean flesh and very sharp teeth.

Source: Lingcod are a northern Pacific fish. In the winter, lingcod are caught off the coast of Alaska. In the summer, lingcod is found off the coast of northern California.

Selection and Handling: Lingcod are sold fresh, frozen and smoked. Smaller lingcod are sold whole or filleted.

Flavor: Mild and delicate.

Flesh: Firm, white with large flakes when cooked.

Preparation: Lingcod steaks and fillets are perfect for grilling and perfect in soups and stews, or pan-fried.

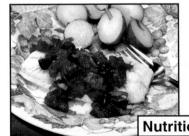

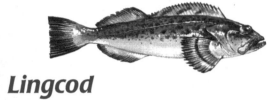

Lingcod

Nutrition Facts		Amount Per 3-Ounce (85-Gram) Serving, (cooked)				
Calories	90	Total Carbohydrate*	0g	0%	Vitamin A*	0%
Calories from Fat	10	Dietary Fiber*	0g	0%	Vitamin C*	0%
Total Fat*	1g	0%	Sugars	0g	Calcium*	0%
Saturated Fat*	0g	0%	Protein	19g	Iron*	0%
Cholesterol*	55mg	20%	Potassium	476mg	* Percent Daily Values are based on a 2,000 calorie diet. Your daily values may be higher or lower, depending on your calorie needs.	
Sodium*	65mg	2%				

Mackerel describes a family of 49 species that includes fish roving in large schools in every ocean and sea of the world.

Source: Chub mackerel are the most popular and are found in warm waters. Atlantic mackerel comes from the mid-Atlantic region of the United States. King mackerel are harvested off South Carolina. Less known species, such as Spanish, wahoo, painted and sierra, are found in the Gulf of Mexico.

Selection and Handling: Since colors fade with age, shop for the most vivid mackerel. Small mackerel weighing about 1 pound (454kg) are sold whole. Larger mackerel are cut into steaks or fillets.

Flavor: Full, distinctive.

Flesh: Moderately firm, few bones.

Preparation: A relatively high oil content makes mackerel perfect for smoking, broiling and grilling.

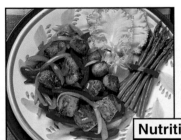

Mackerel, Atlantic/Pacific

Nutrition Facts		Amount Per 3-Ounce (85-Gram) Serving, (cooked)				
Calories	220	Total Carbohydrate*	0g	0%	Vitamin A*	4%
Calories from Fat	140	Dietary Fiber*	0g	0%	Vitamin C*	0%
Total Fat*	15g	25%	Sugars	0g	Calcium*	0%
Saturated Fat*	3.5g	20%	Protein	20g	Iron*	8%
Cholesterol*	65mg	20%	Potassium	341mg	* Percent Daily Values are based on a 2,000 calorie diet. Your daily values may be higher or lower, depending on your calorie needs.	
Sodium*	70mg	2%				

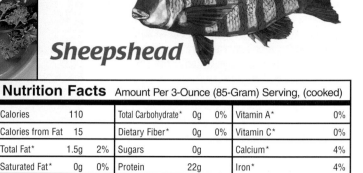
Sheepshead

Sheepshead is a member of the porgy or sea bream family. It has 5 to 7 dark stripes vertically on its sides (hence the common name of convict fish) and strong, unnotched teeth used to eat mollusks and crabs. It is considered a valuable game fish.

Source: Sheepshead are found from Nova Scotia to Florida and around to the Gulf of Mexico. The California Sheepshead is an unrelated species.

Selection and Handling: Market size rarely exceeds 2 pounds (907g). They are sold fresh or frozen as either whole or dressed fish. Rarely they may be found as fillets.

Flavor: Very sweet, said to resemble crabmeat.

Flesh: Lean with a firm flake.

Preparation: The skin of sheepshead may be tough and should be removed prior to cooking. Sheepshead flesh may be steamed, baked, broiled, grilled, fried or roasted.

Nutrition Facts			Amount Per 3-Ounce (85-Gram) Serving, (cooked)				
Calories	110		Total Carbohydrate*	0g	0%	Vitamin A*	0%
Calories from Fat	15		Dietary Fiber*	0g	0%	Vitamin C*	0%
Total Fat*	1.5g	2%	Sugars	0g		Calcium*	4%
Saturated Fat*	0g	0%	Protein	22g		Iron*	4%
Cholesterol*	55mg	20%	Potassium	435mg		* Percent Daily Values are based on a 2,000 calorie diet. Your daily values may be higher or lower, depending on your calorie needs.	
Sodium*	60mg	2%					

Tilapia is also known as St. Peter's fish because biblical scholars believe it to be the fish that St. Peter caught and fed to the multitudes at the Red Sea. Other common names include mouthbrooder and Nile perch.

Source: A native of Africa, tilapia is farm-raised in tropical and temperate climates.

Selection and Handling: Tilapia is sold whole and as fresh or frozen fillets. The color of the meat varies, but pinkish to off-white is most common.

Flavor: Like all farm-raised fish, the flavor depends on the fish's diet and water quality. Tilapia often have a mild, slightly sweet flavor.

Flesh: Moderately firm with tender flakes.

Preparation: Tilapia is excellent baked, broiled, sautéed and grilled. Deep-frying may toughen it. Tilapia is great for showcasing special flavors, such as garlic, dill or lime. It may be used in any recipe calling for flounder or snapper.

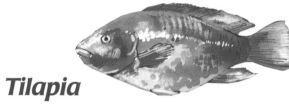
Tilapia

Nutrition Facts			Amount Per 3-Ounce (85-Gram) Serving, (cooked)				
Calories	110		Total Carbohydrate*	0g	0%	Vitamin A*	0%
Calories from Fat	20		Dietary Fiber*	0g	0%	Vitamin C*	2%
Total Fat*	2.5g	4%	Sugars	0g		Calcium*	0%
Saturated Fat*	1g	5%	Protein	22g		Iron*	2%
Cholesterol*	75mg	25%	Potassium	360mg		* Percent Daily Values are based on a 2,000 calorie diet. Your daily values may be higher or lower, depending on your calorie needs.	
Sodium*	30mg	1%					

Rainbow trout is also known as silver trout and brook trout. This fish has a striking appearance, with its heavily spotted body, dark olive-green back, silvery belly and a reddish band (the rainbow) along its side.

Source: Anglers catch wild rainbow trout on four continents, but its sale in the United States is prohibited by law. Nearly every state produces farm-raised trout, however, and Idaho is the undisputed top producer. Farm-raised rainbow trout is available year-round.

Selection and Handling: Rainbow trout is available fresh or frozen as whole, dressed, fillets and steaks. The quality of farm-raised rainbow trout is consistently high.

Flavor: Very mild with a hint of nut-like flavor.

Flesh: Firm with a fairly fine flake.

Preparation: The traditional cookery method for rainbow trout is pan-frying. It is also excellent baked and broiled.

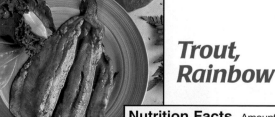

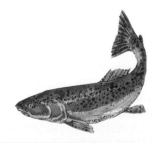
Trout, Rainbow

Nutrition Facts			Amount Per 3-Ounce (85-Gram) Serving, (cooked)				
Calories	140		Total Carbohydrate*	0g	0%	Vitamin A*	4%
Calories from Fat	60		Dietary Fiber*	0g	0%	Vitamin C*	4%
Total Fat*	6g	10%	Sugars	0g		Calcium*	8%
Saturated Fat*	2g	8%	Protein	21g		Iron*	0%
Cholesterol*	60mg	20%	Potassium	375mg		* Percent Daily Values are based on a 2,000 calorie diet. Your daily values may be higher or lower, depending on your calorie needs.	
Sodium*	35mg	0%					

The Dungeness crab, sometimes called the San Francisco crab, is a member of the rock crab family. It has a deep body and heavy carapace, which is usually pinkish green and yellow before cooking and bright red afterward.

Source: Dungeness crabs are harvested from the Aleutians to southern California from November to February.

Selection and Handling: Market forms include precooked whole, dressed sections and picked meat. Out-of-season crabs are sold frozen. Live crabs should be active or move when touched and feel heavy for their size. Do not place live crabs in airtight containers or cover with water. Cook live crabs within 24 hours of purchase.

Flavor: Mild, slightly nutty flavor.

Flesh: Very white, delicately textured.

Preparation: They may be served chilled or reheated by steaming. About 25% of the weight of Dungeness crabs is edible meat.

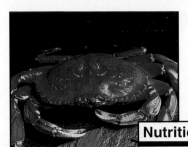

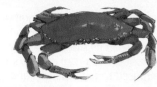

Crab, Dungeness

Nutrition Facts		Amount Per 3-Ounce (85-Gram) Serving, (cooked)			
Calories	90	Total Carbohydrate* <1g	0%	Vitamin A*	0%
Calories from Fat 10		Dietary Fiber* 0g	0%	Vitamin C*	6%
Total Fat*	1g 0%	Sugars 0g		Calcium*	6%
Saturated Fat*	0g 0%	Protein 19g		Iron*	2%
Cholesterol*	65mg 20%	Potassium 347mg		* Percent Daily Values are based on a 2,000 calorie diet. Your daily values may be higher or lower, depending on your calorie needs.	
Sodium*	320mg 15%				

King crab is the largest and most costly of the commercially harvested crabs. Adult king crabs may grow as large as 8 feet (2.4m) across. They have only six legs while most crabs have eight.

Source: King crabs are found in the Arctic waters of the North Pacific. Russia is the top producer, followed by the United States.

Selection and Handling: The most common market size of king crab is 3 to 4 feet (91cm to 1.2m) in diameter and weighing between 4 and 9 pounds (1.8 and 4kg). It is usually sold frozen, as clusters, legs and claws, split legs or picked meat.

Flavor: Distinctively sweet.

Flesh: Succulent and tender, very white with red or orange tinges.

Preparation: King crab is always sold precooked and may be served hot or cold. Heat king crab by broiling or grilling the split legs or by immersing the whole legs or clusters briefly in simmering water.

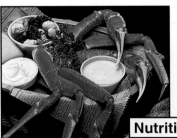

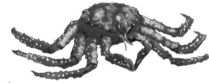

Crab, King

Nutrition Facts		Amount Per 3-Ounce (85-Gram) Serving, (cooked)			
Calories	80	Total Carbohydrate* 0g	0%	Vitamin A*	0%
Calories from Fat 15		Dietary Fiber* 0g	0%	Vitamin C*	10%
Total Fat*	1.5g 2%	Sugars 0g		Calcium*	6%
Saturated Fat*	0g 0%	Protein 16g		Iron*	4%
Cholesterol*	45mg 15%	Potassium 223mg		* Percent Daily Values are based on a 2,000 calorie diet. Your daily values may be higher or lower, depending on your calorie needs.	
Sodium*	910mg 40%				

Snow crab is also known as Tanner crab and queen crab. They are members of the spider crab family with spindly legs and tiny bodies. Snow crabs average 5 pounds (2.3kg) and measure 2 feet (61cm) from tip to tip.

Source: Snow crabs are harvested by Alaskan and Canadian fishermen in the North Pacific and North Atlantic.

Selection and Handling: They are sold precooked and are available as frozen in-shell clusters or, occasionally, as canned meat. Clusters consist of three or four legs, a claw and a shoulder. Clusters should have a fresh smell and should be free of ice crystals and freezer burn. Store frozen for up to six months.

Flavor: Delicate, sweet.

Flesh: Tender, white, moist.

Preparation: Thaw in the refrigerator, never on the counter. Serve cold or reheated by steaming, with melted butter or mustard sauce.

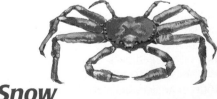

Crab, Snow

Nutrition Facts		Amount Per 3-Ounce (85-Gram) Serving, (cooked)			
Calories	120	Total Carbohydrate* 0g	0%	Vitamin A*	4%
Calories from Fat 50		Dietary Fiber* 0g	0%	Vitamin C*	4%
Total Fat*	5g 8%	Sugars 0g		Calcium*	8%
Saturated Fat*	1g 5%	Protein 16g		Iron*	4%
Cholesterol*	80mg 27%	Potassium 261mg		* Percent Daily Values are based on a 2,000 calorie diet. Your daily values may be higher or lower, depending on your calorie needs.	
Sodium*	270mg 11%				

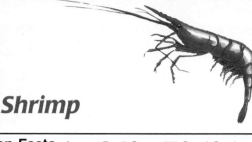

Usually transparent, shrimp can range in color from pink to reddish brown and many shades of green, yellow, brown and gray. The most common commercial shrimp in waters near the United States is the white shrimp. Two other important species are the pink-grooved shrimp and the popular prawn of the Pacific Northwest coast.

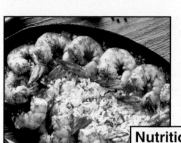

Shrimp

Source: Warm-water shrimp are harvested in tropical waters; cold-water shrimp are found in the Northern Atlantic and Pacific Oceans.

Selection and Handling: Select fresh-smelling shrimp with firm flesh.

Flavor: Mild and sweet; cold-water varieties are sweet tasting.

Flesh: Firm, tender, translucent before cooking.

Preparation: Delicious boiled, fried and grilled.

Nutrition Facts			Amount Per 3-Ounce (85-Gram) Serving, (cooked)				
Calories	80		Total Carbohydrate*	0g	0%	Vitamin A*	4%
Calories from Fat	10		Dietary Fiber*	0g	0%	Vitamin C*	4%
Total Fat*	1g	0%	Sugars	0g		Calcium*	4%
Saturated Fat*	0g	0%	Protein	18g		Iron*	15%
Cholesterol*	166mg	60%	Potassium	155mg		* Percent Daily Values are based on a 2,000 calorie diet. Your daily values may be higher or lower, depending on your calorie needs.	
Sodium*	190mg	8%					

Three species of shrimp provide the majority of landings in the Gulf of Mexico—brown shrimp, white shrimp and pink shrimp.

Source: Gulf shrimp are caught from North Carolina to Mexico, with the heaviest harvest in the summer.

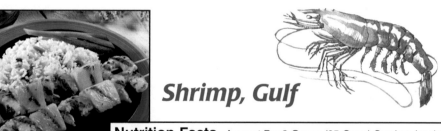

Shrimp, Gulf

Selection and Handling: Shrimp are sized according to the number per pound/kilogram. White shrimp range from 12 to 30 per pound (454g), while brown and pink shrimp range from 16 to 60 per pound (454g). Almost all shrimp are frozen prior to shipping. Most processed shrimp are treated to prevent melanosis (black spot), a natural deterioration of the shell and meat.

Flavor: Sweet, mild.

Flesh: Very firm and tender, ranging from off-white to pink to gray.

Preparation: Shrimp are easier to peel and devein prior to cooking. The sand vein is safe to eat and tasteless, but it may be gritty. Shrimp are especially suited for boiling, frying, stir-frying, sautéing and grilling.

Nutrition Facts			Amount Per 3-Ounce (85-Gram) Serving, (cooked)				
Calories	80		Total Carbohydrate*	0g	0%	Vitamin A*	4%
Calories from Fat	10		Dietary Fiber*	0g	0%	Vitamin C*	4%
Total Fat*	1g	2%	Sugars	0g		Calcium*	4%
Saturated Fat*	0g	0%	Protein	18g		Iron*	15%
Cholesterol*	165mg	55%	Potassium	155mg		* Percent Daily Values are based on a 2,000 calorie diet. Your daily values may be higher or lower, depending on your calorie needs.	
Sodium*	190mg	8%					

Though a member of the shrimp family, rock shrimp could easily be mistaken for a miniature lobster. It has a tough, rigid shell, and it is usually pale pink to reddish-brown.

Source: Rock shrimp is harvested at night from the deep waters of the Gulf of Mexico and the south Atlantic Ocean. Available year-round, it is most abundant in the winter.

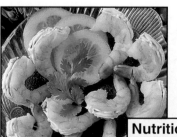
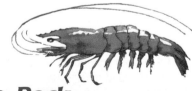

Shrimp, Rock

Selection and Handling: Rock shrimp is usually sold frozen, headless with the shell on or peeled and deveined. There are about 40 shrimp to the pound (454g). Look for a mild, slightly sweet smell and flesh free of discoloration or freezer burn. Use rock shrimp within one day of thawing.

Flavor: Similar to lobster with hints of shrimp.

Flesh: Very firm, like lobster.

Preparation: Before cooking, use kitchen shears to butterfly rock shrimp, then broil or grill. For peeled rock shrimp, simmering is best.

Nutrition Facts			Amount Per 3-Ounce (85-Gram) Serving, (cooked)				
Calories	84		Total Carbohydrate*	0g	0%	Vitamin A*	5%
Calories from Fat	10		Dietary Fiber*	0g	0%	Vitamin C*	4%
Total Fat*	1g	2%	Sugars	0g		Calcium*	4%
Saturated Fat*	0g	0%	Protein	18g		Iron*	15%
Cholesterol*	166mg	54%	Potassium	155mg		* Percent Daily Values are based on a 2,000 calorie diet. Your daily values may be higher or lower, depending on your calorie needs.	
Sodium*	190mg	8%					

Northern or American ("Maine") lobsters are distinguished from other lobsters by a set of claws, one large crusher claw and a smaller one used to hold prey. They can weigh up to 45 pounds (20.5kg), but most are sold at 1 to 5 pounds (454g to 2.3kg).

Source: The lobsters thrive in cold waters of the North Atlantic. They are caught in traps from Labrador down to Virginia.

Selection and Handling: Sold live, frozen, raw or cooked, in shell or out, whole and as picked meat. Look for active live lobsters. Refrigerate live in moist packaging such as seaweed, damp paper strips or cloth for up to 24 hours. Do not place them in airtight containers.

Flavor: Distinctively sweet.

Flesh: Firm, tender, snowy white with red tinges when cooked.

Preparation: Lobsters are best when steamed or boiled. During cooking, greenish-blue live lobsters turn bright red.

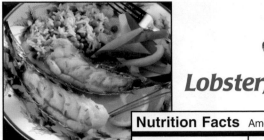

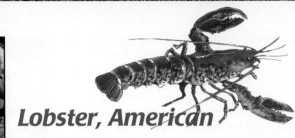

Lobster, American

Nutrition Facts
Amount Per 3-Ounce (85-Gram) Serving, (cooked)

Calories	80	Total Carbohydrate*	0g	0%	Vitamin A*	0%
Calories from Fat	0	Dietary Fiber*	0g	0%	Vitamin C*	0%
Total Fat*	0.5g 0%	Sugars	0g		Calcium*	6%
Saturated Fat*	0g 0%	Protein	17g		Iron*	0%
Cholesterol*	60mg 20%	Potassium	299mg		* Percent Daily Values are based on a 2,000 calorie diet. Your daily values may be higher or lower, depending on your calorie needs.	
Sodium*	320mg 15%					

Also known as rock lobster, spiny lobster is the term applied to over four dozen clawless lobsters. They have short, sharp spines along their bodies and tails. They have green, blue and yellow spots on orange or brown shells.

Source: Spiny lobsters that are found along the Atlantic coast from North Carolina to Brazil are referred to as warm-water lobsters. Those caught off the coasts of South Africa, New Zealand and Australia are known as cold-water lobsters.

Selection and Handling: Primarily, spiny lobsters are marketed as raw or cooked, frozen tails. They are graded by size and prices differ accordingly. Cold-water tails cost more than warm-water tails.

Flavor: Distinctively sweet.

Flesh: Very firm, tender, white with red tinges.

Preparation: Spiny lobster tails can be boiled, steamed or broiled. Baking tends to toughen them.

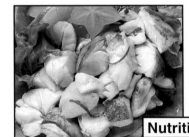

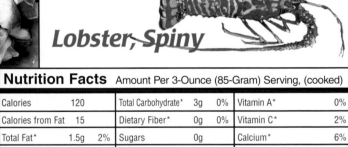

Lobster, Spiny

Nutrition Facts
Amount Per 3-Ounce (85-Gram) Serving, (cooked)

Calories	120	Total Carbohydrate*	3g	0%	Vitamin A*	0%
Calories from Fat	15	Dietary Fiber*	0g	0%	Vitamin C*	2%
Total Fat*	1.5g 2%	Sugars	0g		Calcium*	6%
Saturated Fat*	0g 0%	Protein	22g		Iron*	6%
Cholesterol*	75mg 25%	Potassium	177mg		* Percent Daily Values are based on a 2,000 calorie diet. Your daily values may be higher or lower, depending on your calorie needs.	
Sodium*	190mg 8%					

Surimi, also called imitation crab (or lobster) or mock crab, is a restructured food product made from ground whiting, pollock or other low-priced fish. Flavor concentrate or artificial flavorings are added to fish paste and then formed, cooked, and cut into shapes.

Source: Japanese have been making surimi for centuries. It's also produced in the Northwest coastal areas of North America and Alaska.

Selection and Handling: Look for packaging that is intact with no signs of ice crystals or freezer burn. Keep unopened packages in the refrigerator for up to 2 months or freeze up to 6 months. Once opened, use within 2 to 3 days.

Flavor: Sweet, very similar to king or snow crab.

Flesh: Tender, moist, very white with (artificially colored) red tinges.

Preparation: Imitation crab meat is fully cooked. Use it in any recipe calling for cooked seafood. It's best in salads, casseroles, soups, chowders, spreads or dips.

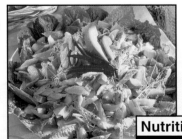

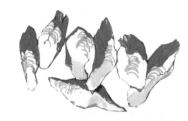

Surimi

Nutrition Facts
Amount Per 3-Ounce (85-Gram) Serving, (cooked)

Calories	90	Total Carbohydrate*	8g	2%	Vitamin A*	0%
Calories from Fat	10	Dietary Fiber*	0g	0%	Vitamin C*	0%
Total Fat*	1.5g 0%	Sugars	0g		Calcium*	0%
Saturated Fat*	0g 0%	Protein	11g		Iron*	2%
Cholesterol*	30mg 10%	Potassium	76mg		* Percent Daily Values are based on a 2,000 calorie diet. Your daily values may be higher or lower, depending on your calorie needs.	
Sodium*	600mg 25%					

Note: Persons with shellfish allergies may be allergic to surimi.

Note: Elderly people, pregnant women, children and people with compromised immune systems should NEVER eat raw shellfish.

Hardshell clams describes many varieties such as quahog, littleneck, top neck, count neck, cherry stone, cockle, chowder, hard, butter, pismo and baby clams.

Source: They are found in both the shallow and deep cool waters of the Atlantic and Pacific oceans. Many farm-raised clams come from the southern United States.

Selection and Handling: Clams must be alive until ready to eat or cook. Look for closed shells or ones that close when tapped. Refrigerate live clams in a bowl, covered with wet paper towels. Never store in airtight containers or cover with plastic wrap. Keep cold, but not on ice.

Flavor: Mild and slightly salty.

Flesh: Somewhat chewy.

Preparation: Scrub the outside of the shells with a stiff brush and cold water before cooking. Clams can be steamed, baked, used in soups, stews or pasta dishes or eaten raw by healthy individuals.

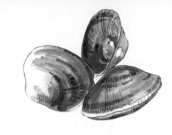

Clams

Nutrition Facts		Amount Per 3-Ounce (85-Gram) Serving, (cooked)			
Calories	130	Total Carbohydrate*	4g 0%	Vitamin A*	10%
Calories from Fat	15	Dietary Fiber*	0g 0%	Vitamin C*	30%
Total Fat*	1.5g 2%	Sugars	0g	Calcium*	8%
Saturated Fat*	0g 0%	Protein	22g	Iron*	130%
Cholesterol*	55mg 20%	Potassium	534mg	* Percent Daily Values are based on a 2,000 calorie diet. Your daily values may be higher or lower, depending on your calorie needs.	
Sodium*	95mg 4%				

Dozens of mussel species are found all over the world. They all have a thin, oblong shell that may be blue, green or yellowish green in color and range from 1½ to 6 inches (3.8 to 15cm) long. The most common is the blue mussel.

Source: They are harvested wild and farm-raised off both coasts of Canada and the United States, as well as in the Mediterranean Sea.

Selection and Handling: Farm-raised mussels have as much as three times the meat of wild mussels. They are harvested year-round, but are most plentiful from October to May. Primarily, they are sold live in net bags. They are also marketed frozen in the shell.

Flavor: Distinctively flavored, somewhat briny.

Flesh: Tender, firm, pinkish in color.

Preparation: Mussels can be eaten raw, by healthy individuals, but are usually cooked. They are often featured a variety of soups and stews or steamed with garlic and butter.

Mussels

Nutrition Facts		Amount Per 3-Ounce (85-Gram) Serving, (cooked)			
Calories	150	Total Carbohydrate*	6g 2%	Vitamin A*	6%
Calories from Fat	35	Dietary Fiber*	0g 0%	Vitamin C*	20%
Total Fat*	4g 6%	Sugars	0g	Calcium*	2%
Saturated Fat*	0.5g 4%	Protein	20g	Iron*	30%
Cholesterol*	50mg 15%	Potassium	228mg	* Percent Daily Values are based on a 2,000 calorie diet. Your daily values may be higher or lower, depending on your calorie needs.	
Sodium*	310mg 15%				

Oysters have hard, rough, gray shells containing meat that varies from beige to gray. Harvested year-round, they are at their best during cold weather.

Source: The Atlantic oyster is harvested along the Atlantic and Gulf of Mexico coasts. The Pacific oyster is harvested primarily in the Pacific Northwest.

Selection and Handling: Shucked oysters should be in a clean liquid. Shell oysters should be tightly closed. Discard any that are open. Never store live oysters in an airtight container or directly on ice.

Flavor: Oysters vary greatly in taste, reflecting the salinity and mineral content of the water from which they were harvested.

Flesh: Texture varies with size and origin.

Preparation: Purists insist that the only way to eat oysters is raw, however, only healthy people should eat raw seafood. Oysters are also delicious fried, baked, broiled, or in a soup or chowder.

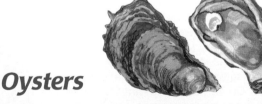

Oysters

Nutrition Facts		Amount Per 3-Ounce (85-Gram) Serving, (cooked)			
Calories	70	Total Carbohydrate*	6g 2%	Vitamin A*	0%
Calories from Fat	15	Dietary Fiber*	0g 0%	Vitamin C*	8%
Total Fat*	2g 2%	Sugars	0g	Calcium*	4%
Saturated Fat*	0.5g 2%	Protein	6g	Iron*	35%
Cholesterol*	30mg 10%	Potassium	129mg	* Percent Daily Values are based on a 2,000 calorie diet. Your daily values may be higher or lower, depending on your calorie needs.	
Sodium*	135mg 6%				

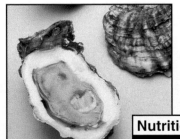

Note: Elderly people, pregnant women, children and people with compromised immune systems should NEVER eat raw shellfish or squid.

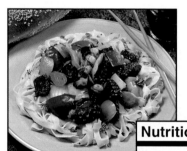

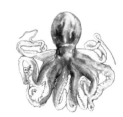

Scallops, Sea

Sea scallops are larger and more widely available than bay scallops. They are about 1½ inches (3.8cm) in diameter and slightly less tender than smaller scallops.

Source: Most sea scallops are harvested by dredges and are found from Newfoundland to North Carolina. Pacific sea scallops are found from Alaska to Oregon. Scallops are usually shucked and chilled or frozen onboard ship.

Selection and Handling: Look for scallops with an ivory or pinkish color and firm meat. They should be free of excessive amounts of liquid or objectionable odor. "Soakers" are scallops that have been over-treated with phosphates, giving them a rubbery texture and chalky white color.

Flavor: Distinctively sweet with hints of nuts.

Flesh: Lean, firm and tender.

Preparation: Bake, fry, poach, sauté, grill or broil. Cook until opaque. Do not overcook. Cooking time depends on size and cooking method.

Nutrition Facts		Amount Per 3-Ounce (85-Gram) Serving, (cooked)			
Calories	180	Total Carbohydrate*	9g	2%	Vitamin A*	0%
Calories from Fat	90	Dietary Fiber*	0g	0%	Vitamin C*	4%
Total Fat*	9g	15%	Sugars	0g	Calcium*	4%
Saturated Fat*	2.5g	10%	Protein	15g	Iron*	4%
Cholesterol*	50mg	15%	Potassium	283mg	* Percent Daily Values are based on a 2,000 calorie diet. Your daily values may be higher or lower, depending on your calorie needs.
Sodium*	390mg	15%			

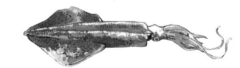

Octopus

The U.S. imports octopi from around the world. They can be as small as 1 inch (2.5cm) or grow to over 6 feet (1.8m). Most weigh 3 pounds (1.36kg) and are only 1 to 2 feet (30.5 to 61cm) in length, with tentacles extended.

Source: Octopi are found worldwide.

Selection and Handling: Fresh octopi are available on the East Coast in November and December. They are generally sold already cleaned.

Flavor: Mild but flavorful.

Flesh: It appears bluish-gray until cooked, then skin turns purplish and the inner flesh a pure white. The texture is firm to chewy.

Preparation: Turn the head inside out, like a sock. Carefully remove the ink sac under running water. Turn the octopus right side out and cut off the part where the eyes are. Larger, older octopus is best simmered in liquid for 1 hour or until tender.

Nutrition Facts		Amount Per 3-Ounce (85-Gram) Serving, (cooked)			
Calories	140	Total Carbohydrate*	4g	1%	Vitamin A*	6%
Calories from Fat	15	Dietary Fiber*	0g	0%	Vitamin C*	10%
Total Fat*	2g	3%	Sugars	0g	Calcium*	10%
Saturated Fat*	0g	0%	Protein	25g	Iron*	45%
Cholesterol*	80mg	27%	Potassium	535mg	* Percent Daily Values are based on a 2,000 calorie diet. Your daily values may be higher or lower, depending on your calorie needs.
Sodium*	390mg	16%			

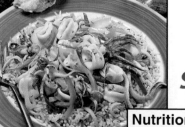

Squid/Calamari

Squid are also known as calamari or inkfish.

Source: Squid are caught in the Atlantic and Pacific oceans, as well as the Mediterranean Sea. The greatest supply comes from Japan, Argentina and Morocco. In North America, summer squid are harvested from Canada's Atlantic Ocean waters and winter squid from the Atlantic waters near the United States.

Selection and Handling: Squid are available fresh or frozen, whole and cleaned in rings or steaks. Color ranges from purple to white. Avoid brown-colored squid or frozen squid with freezer burn.

Flavor: Delicate, slightly sweet.

Flesh: Very firm, somewhat chewy, very white when cooked.

Preparation: Both tentacles and the body (often cut into rings) are used. Fried squid is a favorite hors d'oeuvre. Calamari is often not cooked, but is marinated in a citrus-based dressing. For stuffed squid, leave the body intact and stuff with vegetables before baking.

Nutrition Facts		Amount Per 3-Ounce (85-Gram) Serving, (cooked)			
Calories	150	Total Carbohydrate*	7g	2%	Vitamin A*	0%
Calories from Fat	60	Dietary Fiber*	0g	0%	Vitamin C*	6%
Total Fat*	6g	10%	Sugars	0g	Calcium*	4%
Saturated Fat*	1.5g	8%	Protein	15g	Iron*	4%
Cholesterol*	221mg	70%	Potassium	237mg	* Percent Daily Values are based on a 2,000 calorie diet. Your daily values may be higher or lower, depending on your calorie needs.
Sodium*	260mg	10%			

meat and seafood recipes

Steak de Burgo

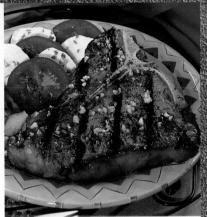

2   tbsp. (30ml) chopped fresh basil or 1½ tsp. (7.5ml) dried basil
4   tsp. (20ml) olive oil
2   cloves garlic, chopped
2   (1-lb./454g) beef T-bone steaks, cut 1 inch (2.54cm) thick
Freshly ground black pepper

1. Preheat grill to medium. In a small bowl stir together basil, olive oil and garlic. Rub over both sides of steaks. Season steaks with pepper.
2. Grill directly for 11 to 14 minutes for medium rare or 14 to 16 minutes for medium, turning once.

Serves 4

Individual Beef Wellingtons

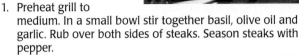

4   (3-oz./85g) beef tenderloin fillets, 1 inch (2.54cm) thick
¼   tsp. (1ml) salt
¼   tsp. (1ml) pepper
2   tbsp. (30ml) butter or margarine
1   (8-oz./227g) pkg. sliced fresh mushrooms
1   shallot, finely chopped
2   tbsp. (30ml) beef broth
½   tsp. dried Italian seasoning
1   (17¼-oz./489g) pkg. frozen puff pastry sheets, thawed
1   egg white, lightly beaten

1. Sprinkle beef with salt and pepper. Melt butter in a large skillet over medium heat; add beef and cook 3 minutes on each side or until browned. Remove from skillet and let cool.
2. Add mushrooms and shallots; sauté 5 minutes. Stir in beef broth and Italian seasoning.
3. Unfold one pastry sheet on a lightly floured surface; roll out to 12x12-inch (30.5x30.5cm) square. Cut pastry into four squares. Place one fillet in center of each square; top with mushroom mixture. Bring opposite corners together over beef, gently pressing to seal. Place on a baking sheet and brush lightly with beaten egg white.
4. Bake at 425°F (218°C) on the lowest oven rack for 20 to 25 minutes or until golden and meat thermometer registers 160°F (71°C).

Serves 4

Sirloin Steak Salad

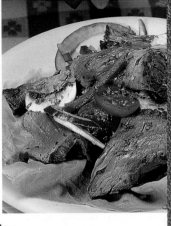

1   (12-oz./340g) beef top sirloin steak, 1 inch (2.54cm) thick
2   cups (473ml) cherry tomatoes, halved
1   medium red onion, peeled and thinly sliced
1   medium red bell pepper, julienned
1   cup (237ml) sliced mushrooms
¼   cup (59ml) chopped fresh chives
3   tbsp. (44ml) chopped fresh parsley
¼   cup (59ml) Italian fat free or low-calorie salad dressing
6   cups (1.4l) assorted greens

1. Preheat grill to medium. Season steak with salt and pepper.
2. Grill steak to desired doneness (14 to 18 minutes for medium rare, 18 to 22 minutes for medium), turning once. Cool 10 minutes.
3. Thinly slice steak on the diagonal. Combine steak, tomatoes, onion, bell pepper, mushrooms, chives and parsley. Drizzle with dressing; toss to coat. Serve on lettuce leaves.

Serves 4

Sweet-and-Sour Chuck Roast

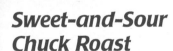

½   tsp. (2.5ml) salt
½   tsp. (2.5ml) pepper
1   (3-lb./1.36kg) boneless chuck roast, trimmed
1   tbsp. (15ml) vegetable oil
2   cloves garlic, minced
2   tbsp. (30ml) firmly packed dark brown sugar
1   cup (237ml) ketchup
1   (12-oz./340g) bottle chili sauce
¼   cup (59ml) red wine vinegar
2   medium onions, thinly sliced

1. Sprinkle salt and pepper evenly over roast. Brown roast 2 minutes on each side in hot oil in a Dutch oven over medium-high heat.
2. Stir together garlic, sugar, ketchup, chili sauce and vinegar. Pour over roast. Add onions.
3. Bake, covered, at 350°F (177°C) for 2½ to 3 hours, or until tender and meat thermometer registers 160°F (71°C).

Serves 4 to 6

Beef Stroganoff

2 lb. (907g) beef stew meat
1 tbsp. (15ml) vegetable oil
1 (8-oz./227g) pkg. sliced fresh mushrooms
1 (10¾-oz./305g) can Cream of Mushroom Soup
1 (10¾-oz./305g) can Cream of Celery Soup
1 (1.25-oz./35g) pkg. onion soup mix
6 cups (1.4l) dried egg noodles (12 oz./340g)
Dairy sour cream (optional)

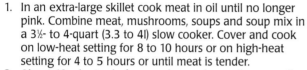

1. In an extra-large skillet cook meat in oil until no longer pink. Combine meat, mushrooms, soups and soup mix in a 3½- to 4-quart (3.3 to 4l) slow cooker. Cover and cook on low-heat setting for 8 to 10 hours or on high-heat setting for 4 to 5 hours or until meat is tender.
2. About 10 minutes before serving cook noodles according to package directions. Serve stroganoff over noodles. Serve with a dollop of sour cream, if desired.
Serves 6

Blue Cheese and Bacon Burgers

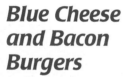

1 lb. (454g) lean ground beef
8 slices thick sliced bacon, crisp-cooked and drained
½ tsp. (2.5ml) coarse ground black pepper
½ cup (118ml) crumbled blue cheese
4 Kaiser rolls, split
Lettuce leaves (optional)
Tomato slices (optional)
Onion slices (optional)

1. Shape beef into four ¾-inch (1.9cm) thick patties. Grill patties on the rack of an uncovered grill over medium coals for 14 to 18 minutes or until done (160°F/71°C).
2. Place two bacon pieces on each burger. Sprinkle with pepper. Top with blue cheese. Grill about 2 minutes more or until cheese begins to melt. Serve on rolls with lettuce, tomato, and onion, if desired.
Serves 4

Baked Brisket

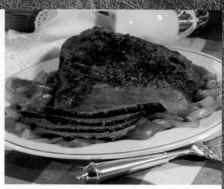

2 large onions
1 3- to 3½-lb. (1.36 to 1.58kg) beef brisket
3 tbsp. (44ml) barbecue seasoning or Caribbean jerk seasoning

1. Preheat oven to 325°F (163°C). Cut onions into ½-inch (1.3cm) slices. Place in the bottom of 13x9x2-inch baking pan. Trim fat from meat. Rub seasoning over all sides of meat. Place meat in baking pan.
2. Cover pan with foil. Bake about 3 hours or until meat is tender.
3. To serve, thinly slice meat and serve with onions and juices.
Serves 10 to 12

Italian Pot Roast

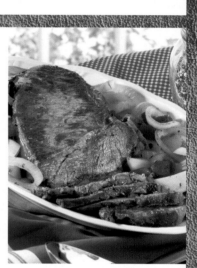

1 2- to 3-lb. (907g to 1.36kg) boneless beef chuck pot roast
2 tbsp. (44ml) vegetable oil
3 medium potatoes, peeled and cut into 1-inch (2.54cm) pieces
1 medium onion, sliced
1 (14½ oz./411g) can diced tomatoes
1 tbsp. (15ml) Worcestershire sauce
1 tsp. (5ml) rosemary leaves
1 tsp. (5ml) oregano leaves
1 tsp. (5ml) basil leaves
1 tsp. (5ml) ground black pepper
½ cup (118ml) cold water
⅓ cup (79ml) flour

1. Trim fat from meat. If necessary, cut meat to fit a 5- to 6-quart (4.73 to 5.68l) crockery cooker. In a large skillet quickly brown meat on both sides in hot cooking oil.
2. Place potatoes and onion in the crockery cooker. Top with meat. Stir together undrained tomatoes, Worcestershire sauce, rosemary, oregano, basil and pepper. Pour over meat. Cover and cook on low heat setting for 8 to 10 hours.
3. Remove meat and vegetables from crockery cooker. Keep warm. Measure juices; skim fat. If necessary, add enough water to juices to equal 1¾ cups (415ml).
4. Pour juices into a small saucepan. Stir together water and flour. Stir into juices. Cook and stir until mixture comes to a boil and thickens. Season to taste with salt and pepper. Serve over meat and vegetables.
Serves 6

Veal Chops with Tarragon

4   veal loin chops,
    ¾ inch (1.9cm) thick
1   tbsp. (15ml) chopped
    fresh tarragon, divided
1   tsp. (5ml) kosher salt
¼   tsp. (1ml) pepper
½   cup (118ml) chicken
    broth

1. Trim fat from veal chops. Combine 1½ teaspoons (7.5ml) of the tarragon, salt and pepper. Rub veal with tarragon mixture.
2. Spray large nonstick skillet with nonstick cooking spray and heat over medium heat. Add veal chops and cook for 6 to 8 minutes or until chops are slightly pink in the center, turning once. Remove chops; keep warm.
3. For sauce, add broth to skillet, stirring to scrape up any browned bits. Bring to a boil. Cook until liquid is reduced by half. Stir in remaining 1½ teaspoons (7.5ml) tarragon.
4. Spoon sauce over chops. Garnish with additional fresh tarragon, if desired.
Serves 4

Osso Buco

4   (10-oz./284g) veal shanks
    (1½ inches/3.81cm thick)
1   tsp. (5ml) salt
1   tsp. (5ml) pepper
2   tbsp. (30ml) olive oil
1   large onion, diced
1   cup (237ml) diced carrots
1   cup (237ml) chopped
    celery
2   cloves garlic, minced
1   cup (237ml) dry white wine
1   (14½-oz./411g) can diced
    tomatoes, undrained
1   (10½-oz./298g) can beef broth
¼   cup (59ml) chopped fresh parsley

1. Season veal with salt and pepper. Heat olive oil over medium-high heat in heavy skillet and sear veal shanks 2 minutes on each side or until browned. Remove veal from skillet and place in a lightly greased ovenproof dish. Reduce heat; add onion, carrots, celery and garlic to skillet. Cook, stirring often, for 5 minutes. Add wine, tomatoes and beef broth; bring to a boil and simmer for 5 minutes. Pour over veal.
2. Bake, covered, at 350°F (177°C) for 1 hour and 30 minutes or until veal is tender and a meat thermometer registers 160°F (71°C) . Sprinkle with fresh parsley and serve with broth mixture.
Serves 6

Italian Veal Scallopini

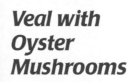

⅓   cup (79ml) Italian seasoned
    bread crumbs
¼   tsp. (1ml) pepper
1   lb. (454g) veal scallopini
2   tbsp. (30ml) olive oil
½   cup (118ml) white wine
3   tbsp. (44ml) lemon juice
1   tsp. (5ml) butter or
    margarine
2   tbsp. (30ml) capers
2   tbsp. (30ml) fresh parsley
Additional fresh parsley and
    lemon slices (optional)

1. Combine bread crumbs and pepper in a small bowl; dredge veal in bread crumb mixture.
2. Heat olive oil in a large skillet over medium-high heat; add veal and cook 1 to 2 minutes on each side or until golden. Remove from skillet and keep warm.
3. Add wine, lemon juice and butter to skillet, stirring to loosen browned particles. Cook until thoroughly heated. Stir in capers and parsley; spoon over veal and serve. Garnish with fresh parsley and lemon slices, if desired.
Serves 4

Veal with Oyster Mushrooms

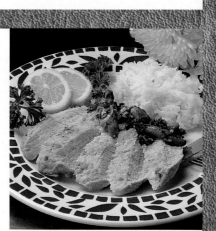

4   veal cutlets, ¼ inch
    (.64cm) thick
½   cup (118ml) flour
2   tbsp. (30ml) butter
1½ cups (355ml) fresh
    oyster mushrooms,
    halved
3   green onions, chopped
1   tbsp. (15ml) chopped
    fresh parsley
½   cup (118ml) beef broth
4   tsp. (20ml) fresh lemon juice

1. Coat veal with flour. Melt butter in large skillet over medium-high heat. Add veal and cook 3 minutes. Turn over. Cook 2 to 3 minutes more or until juices run clear. Season with salt and pepper.
2. Remove meat; keep warm. Add mushrooms, green onions and parsley to skillet. Cook for 3 to 4 minutes or until tender.
3. Add beef broth. Bring to a boil. Cook until reduced by half. Stir in lemon juice. Spoon mushroom mixture over cutlets.
Serves 4

Veal Cutlets with Herb Crust

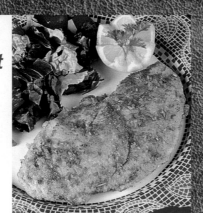

2   (4-oz./113g) veal cutlets
½   cup (118ml) flour
1   egg, beaten
1   cup (237ml) fresh bread crumbs
¼   tsp. (1ml) chopped fresh parsley
¼   tsp. (1ml) chopped fresh chives
1   tbsp. (15ml) butter
2   tbsp. (30ml) lemon juice

1. Place veal between 2 sheets of waxed paper. Using the flat side of a meat mallet, pound veal until ¼ inch (.64cm) thick. Remove waxed paper.
2. Coat veal with flour; dip in beaten egg. Combine bread crumbs, parsley and chives. Dip veal in crumb mixture.
3. In large skillet cook veal in butter over medium heat for 2 to 3 minutes or until juices run clear, turning once. Remove veal to serving plates. Stir lemon juice into drippings in skillet. Pour lemon mixture over veal. Sprinkle with additional chopped chives, if desired.

Serves 2

Veal Chops Porcini

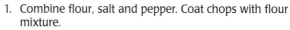

¼   cup (59ml) flour
½   tsp. (2.5ml) salt
¼   tsp. (1ml) pepper
4   veal loin chops, 1 inch (2.54cm) thick
4   tbsp. (59ml) butter
1   lb. (454g) fresh porcini mushrooms, chopped
2   tbsp. (30ml) chopped fresh parsley
1   tsp. (5ml) toasted sesame oil

1. Combine flour, salt and pepper. Coat chops with flour mixture.
2. In a large skillet melt half of the butter over medium heat. Add chops and cook for 5 minutes; turn chops over. Cook 4 to 5 minutes more or until slightly pink in center. Remove chops; keep warm.
3. Melt remaining butter in same skillet; add mushrooms; cook about 5 minutes or until tender. Stir in parsley and sesame oil.
4. Serve mushroom mixture over chops.

Serves 4

Veal Scallopini Piccata with Almonds

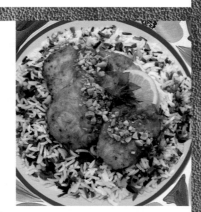

1¼ lb. (567g) veal scallopini
½   cup (118ml) flour
1   tbsp. (15ml) olive oil
1   tbsp. (15ml) butter
¼   cup (59ml) dry white wine
1   tbsp. (30ml) fresh lemon juice
1   tbsp. (30ml) chopped fresh parsley
¼   cup (59ml) chopped almonds, toasted

1. Coat veal with flour, shaking off excess. In large skillet heat oil and butter over high heat. Add half of the veal. Cook for 2 to 3 minutes or until juices run clear, turning once. Season with salt and pepper. Remove veal to platter; keep warm. Repeat with remaining veal.
2. For sauce, add wine and lemon juice to skillet. Bring to a boil, stirring to scrape up browned bits. Stir in parsley. Ladle sauce over veal; sprinkle with almonds.

Serves 4

Veal in Mustard Cream Sauce

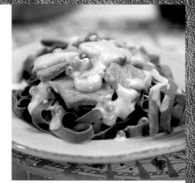

1   (12-oz./340g) pkg. refrigerated spinach fettuccine
1   lb. (454g) veal cutlets, cut ¼-inch (.64cm) thick
4   tsp. (20ml) butter or margarine, divided
1⅓ cups (316ml) reduced-sodium chicken broth
⅔   cup (158ml) fat-free half-and-half or milk
¼   cup (59ml) Dijon-style mustard
2   tbsp. (30ml) flour
2   tbsp. (30ml) capers

1. Cook fettuccine according to package directions; drain.
2. Cut veal into 2-inch (5.08cm) pieces. In a large skillet cook half of veal in half of butter or margarine for 2 to 3 minutes or until juices run clear. Remove from skillet; keep warm. Repeat with remaining veal and butter.
3. Stir chicken broth into drippings in skillet. Cook over high heat for 5 to 8 minutes or until reduced by half. Meanwhile, in a small bowl stir together half-and-half, mustard and flour. Stir into mixture in skillet. Cook and stir until mixture comes to a boil. Stir in capers.
4. Serve veal on top of fettuccine. Spoon sauce over all. Sprinkle with pepper, if desired.

Serves 4

Maple Mustard Pork Chops

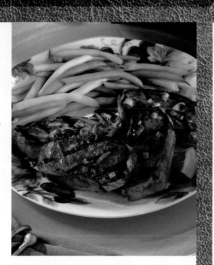

4   boneless pork loin chops, cut 1 inch (2.54cm) thick
3   tbsp. (44ml) Dijon-style mustard
2   tbsp. (30ml) maple syrup
2   tbsp. (30ml) sliced green onion
2   tsp. (10ml) finely shredded orange peel

1. Preheat grill to medium. Trim fat from chops, if necessary. Generously season with pepper.
2. In a small bowl stir together mustard, syrup, onion and orange peel. Set aside.
3. Grill chops 12 to 15 minutes or until juices run clear (160°F/71°C), turning once and brushing with mustard mixture during the last 5 minutes of grilling.

Serves 4

Ham with Chutney Sauce

1   clove garlic
1   small onion, sliced
1   (9-oz./255g) jar mango chutney
3   tbsp. (44ml) Dijon-style mustard
3   tbsp. (44ml) fresh orange juice
¼   cup (59ml) light brown sugar
½   tsp. (2.5ml) ground cloves
1   (7- to 8-lb./3.18 to 3.64kg) fully cooked, spiral-cut ham

1. Add garlic, onion, chutney, mustard, juice, sugar and cloves in a food processor and process until smooth.
2. Place ham in a heavy roasting pan. Pour glaze over ham. Bake at 350°F (177°C) for 1 hour and 30 minutes or until ham is golden brown and a meat thermometer registers 140°F (60°C).

Serves 16

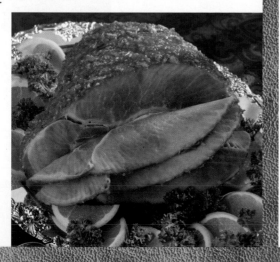

Seasoned Pork Loin

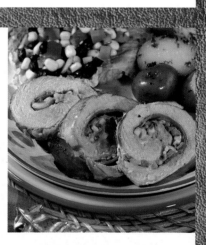

3- to 4-lb. (1.36kg to 1.82kg) pork loin roast
1   large onion, sliced
1   bag (1 lb./454g) baby carrots
3   garlic cloves, minced
2   tsp. (10ml) seasoned salt
½   tsp. (2.5ml) lemon pepper seasoning salt

1. Preheat oven to 325°F (163°C). Place pork roast in a shallow pan. Place sliced onion and carrots around tenderloin. Sprinkle garlic and seasoning salts over top.
2. Cover tightly with foil. Bake for 1¾ to 2½ hours or until an instant read thermometer inserted in center of meat registers 160°F (71°C).

Serves 12

Bacon and Mushroom Stuffed Pork Tenderloin

1   (12-oz./340g) pork tenderloin
2   tsp. (10ml) prepared horseradish
4   slices turkey bacon
½   cup (118ml) finely chopped fresh mushrooms
⅓   cup (79ml) finely chopped onion
1   tsp. (5ml) bottled minced garlic
Vegetable oil

1. Using a sharp knife, make a lengthwise cut down center of tenderloin, cutting to but not through the opposite side. Spread meat open. Place meat between 2 pieces of plastic wrap. Working from the center to the edges, use the flat side of a meat mallet to pound meat into a 10-inch (25.4cm) square. Remove plastic wrap. Spread horseradish evenly over meat.
2. In a large skillet cook bacon until done but not crisp. Drain on paper towels, reserving drippings in skillet. Cook mushrooms, onion and garlic in hot drippings until tender. Arrange bacon slices on meat. Sprinkle mushroom mixture over bacon. Roll up meat. Tie with 100% cotton string at 1-inch (2.54cm) intervals. Brush all surfaces of meat with a little oil.
3. Preheat grill to medium hot and prepare for indirect cooking. Grill tenderloin, covered, for 40 to 50 minutes or until done (160°F/71°C).

Serves 4

Grilled Ham with Summer Fruit Sauce

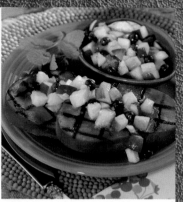

1   1-inch-thick (2.54cm), fully cooked ham slice (about 1½ lb./680g)
1   cup (237ml) pineapple chunks
1   nectarine, sliced or 1 peach, peeled and sliced
¼   cup (59ml) orange marmalade
1   cup (237ml) blueberries or 1 dark sweet cherries, halved and pitted

1. Preheat grill to medium. Place ham on grill and cook for 10 minutes. Meanwhile, for fruit sauce, in a foil pan stir together pineapple, nectarines and marmalade.
2. Turn ham and place fruit on grill beside ham. Cook 10 to 12 minutes more or until ham is heated through and fruit is warm. Remove from grill. Stir blueberries into warm fruit.
3. Cut ham into serving-size pieces. Serve warm fruit sauce with ham.

Serves 6

Brown Sugar Pork Tenderloin

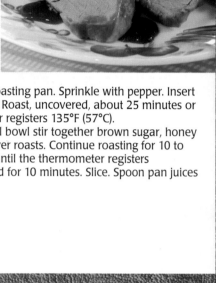

2   (1-lb./454g) pork tenderloins
1   cup (237ml) packed brown sugar
¼   cup (59ml) honey
¼   cup (59ml) prepared mustard

1. Preheat oven to 425°F (218°C). Place pork tenderloins on a rack in a shallow roasting pan. Sprinkle with pepper. Insert a meat thermometer. Roast, uncovered, about 25 minutes or until the thermometer registers 135°F (57°C).
2. Meanwhile, in a small bowl stir together brown sugar, honey and mustard. Pour over roasts. Continue roasting for 10 to 15 minutes more or until the thermometer registers 160°F (71°C). Let stand for 10 minutes. Slice. Spoon pan juices over meat.

Serves 8

Sausage & Bacon Kabobs

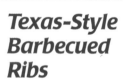

1   cup (237ml) dried apricot halves (about 24 halves)
1   lb. (454g) Italian sausage links
8   slices thick sliced bacon
⅓   cup (79ml) apricot preserves
2   tbsp. (30ml) Dijon-style mustard
2   tsp. (10ml) Worcestershire sauce
    Hot cooked rice (optional)

1. Soak apricot halves in enough warm water to cover for 10 minutes. Drain. Set aside.
2. Use a fork to pierce several holes in skin of each sausage link. In a large saucepan combine sausages and enough water to cover. Bring to a boil; reduce heat. Simmer, uncovered, for 10 minutes. Drain. Cool slightly. Cut into ¾-inch-thick (1.9cm) slices.
3. In a large skillet cook bacon until nearly done, but not crisp. Drain on paper towels. On eight long skewers, alternately thread apricot halves and sausage slices, weaving bacon back and forth between them.
4. In a small bowl stir together preserves, mustard and Worcestershire sauce. Grill kabobs over medium-hot coals for 8 to 10 minutes or until heated through, turning and brushing with apricot mixture occasionally. Serve on hot cooked rice, if desired.

Serves 6

Texas-Style Barbecued Ribs

3   to 4 lb. (1.36 to 1.82kg) pork spareribs
2   medium onions, cut into wedges
1   tsp. (5ml) salt
1   tsp. (5ml) ground black pepper
1   tsp. (5ml) dried oregano leaves
1   (18 oz./511g) bottle barbecue sauce

1. Cut ribs into serving-size pieces. Place ribs, onions, salt, pepper and oregano in a 4- to 6-quart (3.8 to 5.68l) Dutch oven. Add enough water to cover. Bring to a boil; reduce heat. Cover and simmer about 1 hour or until ribs are tender; drain.
2. Preheat oven to 350°F (177°C). Brush some of the barbecue sauce over both sides of ribs. Place ribs, bone side down, in a shallow roasting pan. Bake, uncovered, about 30 minutes or until glazed and heated through.
3. Meanwhile, in a small saucepan heat the remaining sauce. Pass sauce with ribs.

Serves 4 to 6

Apricot-Glazed Turkey with Vegetable Stuffing

1 (12-lb./5.46kg) turkey, thawed
1 tsp. (5ml) salt
¾ tsp. (4ml) pepper
Vegetable Stuffing (see recipe below)
1 (14½-oz./411g) can chicken broth
1 cup (237ml) apricot preserves
¼ cup (59ml) fresh orange juice
2 tbsp. (30ml) honey
1 tsp. (5ml) grated orange rind
¼ tsp. (1ml) paprika

Vegetable Stuffing
¼ to ½ cup (59 to 118ml) butter or margarine
2 large celery ribs, diced
1 medium onion, diced
2 parsnips, diced
2 cups (473ml) chopped kale
1 (16-oz./454g) pkg. herb-seasoned stuffing mix (4 cups/.95l)
1 (14½-oz./411g) can chicken broth

1. Remove giblets and neck from turkey, and reserve for another use. Rinse turkey with cold water and pat dry.
2. Sprinkle turkey cavity with salt and pepper. Spoon Vegetable Stuffing into turkey cavity. Place turkey, breast side up, in a large greased roasting pan. Tuck wings under; wrap ends of legs with aluminum foil. Pour chicken broth in bottom of pan.
3. Stir together preserves and next 3 ingredients in a small saucepan. Cook over medium heat, stirring constantly, 5 minutes or until preserves are melted.
4. Brush top of turkey generously with preserves mixture. Sprinkle with paprika.
5. Bake on lowest oven rack at 350°F (177°C) for 3 hours, basting occasionally with preserves mixture. Reduce oven temperature to 325°F (163°C), and bake 30 minutes more or until a meat thermometer inserted into thigh registers 180°F (82°C), basting occasionally. Cover with aluminum foil to prevent excessive browning, if necessary. Let stand 10 minutes before slicing.

Vegetable Stuffing
1. Melt butter in a Dutch oven over medium heat; add next 4 ingredients and sauté 5 to 7 minutes or until tender. Stir in remaining ingredients. Let cool slightly.
Serves 12

Citrus-Herb Turkey

1 (6-lb./2.7kg) turkey breast
1 tbsp. (15ml) butter or margarine, melted
2 tbsp. (30ml) chopped fresh rosemary
2 tbsp. (30ml) chopped fresh sage
2 oranges, thinly sliced
2 lemons, thinly sliced
1 large onion, quartered
2 cups (473ml) chicken broth

1. Salt and pepper turkey to taste.
2. Stir together butter, rosemary and sage. Loosen skin from turkey without detaching and spread half of butter mixture under skin. Arrange one quarter of the orange and lemon slices over butter mixture. Gently pull skin over fruit.
3. Place turkey in a foil-lined pan coated with cooking spray. Place remaining fruit slices, onion and chicken broth in pan. Pour remaining butter-herb mixture over turkey.
4. Bake turkey at 325°F (163°C) for 1 hour and 30 minutes. Cover loosely with foil and bake 1 more hour or until meat thermometer inserted in thickest portion registers 180°F (82°C), basting every 30 minutes. Let stand 10 minutes before serving. Serve with pan juices. Garnish with fresh rosemary, if desired.
Serves 8

Duck with Chestnuts

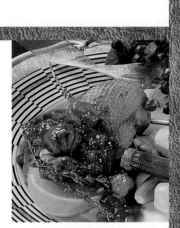

1 large duck
2 large oranges
1 onion, finely chopped
1 lb. (454g) chestnuts
2 sprigs fresh thyme
1 tbsp. (15ml) red currant jelly

1. Cut duck into 2 breast pieces and 4 leg and thigh pieces or have the butcher do it for you. Make strong stock with back, neck and wings.
2. Heat a large skillet to hot and sauté duck pieces until golden on all sides.
3. Remove duck and pour off all but 1 tablespoon of fat and gently fry a finely chopped large onion until golden.
4. Grate orange rind and juice 2 large oranges. Add zest and juice to deglaze the pan.
5. Add duck legs, thighs and fresh thyme and enough stock to cover. Simmer 30 minutes.
6. Meanwhile, peel and parboil chestnuts. Add chestnuts and breasts to pan and cook 20 minutes.
7. Remove duck and chestnuts. Boil sauce until reduced and add jelly. Pour over duck and serve.
Serves 4

Raspberry-Glazed Turkey Tenderloins

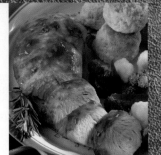

1   cup (237ml) seedless raspberry preserves
½   cup (118ml) light soy sauce
¼   cup (59ml) olive oil
2   cloves garlic, minced
2   tbsp. (30ml) grated fresh gingerroot
1½ tsp. (7.5ml) chopped fresh rosemary (optional)
6   (¾-lb./340g) turkey tenderloins

1. Whisk together preserves, soy sauce, oil, garlic and gingerroot, and chopped rosemary, if desired. Reserve ½ cup (118ml) of the marinade. Place turkey in a heavy-duty resealable plastic bag; pour remaining marinade over turkey. Seal and refrigerate 8 hours, turning occasionally.
2. Remove turkey from marinade, discarding marinade. Arrange turkey on a rack in a broiler pan coated with cooking spray.
3. Bake at 425°F (218°C) for 25 to 35 minutes or until a meat thermometer registers 170°F (77°C), basting often with reserved marinade. Let stand 5 minutes before slicing. Cut into ½-inch-thick (1.27cm) slices for main dish servings or ½-inch-thick (1.27cm) slices for appetizer servings. Garnish with fresh rosemary sprigs, if desired.
Serves 6

Stuffed Cornish Game Hens

6   (1½-lb./680g) Cornish hens
1   tbsp. (15ml) poultry seasoning
1   tsp. (5ml) salt
1   tsp. (5ml) freshly ground pepper
12 prunes, pitted and chopped
3   apples, cored, peeled and diced
1   onion, chopped
1   cup (237ml) apricot preserves
⅓   cup (79ml) white wine
¼   cup (59ml) butter

1. Rub hens with poultry seasoning, salt and pepper; set aside. Spoon prunes, apples and onion evenly into each hen cavity; tie legs together. Place hens on a rack of an aluminum foil-lined roasting pan.
2. Stir together preserves, wine and butter in a small saucepan. Cook over medium heat, stirring constantly, 5 minutes or until preserves are melted.
3. Brush hens with apricot mixture and bake at 350°F (177°C) for 1 hour, basting occasionally. Cover loosely with foil and bake 30 minutes more or until a meat thermometer registers 180°F (82°C).
Serves 6

Champagne Chicken

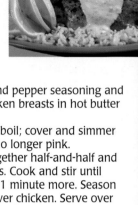

4   boneless, skinless chicken breast halves
Lemon and pepper seasoning salt
Garlic salt
1   tbsp. (15ml) butter or margarine
1   cup (237ml) champagne or reduced-sodium chicken broth
1   cup (237ml) half-and-half or light cream
2   tbsp. (30ml) flour

1. Season chicken lightly with lemon and pepper seasoning and garlic salt. In large skillet brown chicken breasts in hot butter about 2 minutes per side.
2. Add champagne or broth. Bring to a boil; cover and simmer 10 to 12 minutes or until chicken is no longer pink.
3. Remove chicken; keep warm. Stir together half-and-half and flour. Stir flour mixture into pan juices. Cook and stir until thickened and bubbly. Cook and stir 1 minute more. Season with salt and pepper. Spoon sauce over chicken. Serve over parsleyed rice and garnish with lemon slices, if desired.
Serves 4

Lemon-Thyme Roasted Chicken

1   (5-lb./2.27kg) roasting chicken
⅓   cup (79ml) olive oil, divided
1½ tsp. (7.5ml) kosher salt, divided
1½ tsp. (7.5ml) cracked black pepper, divided
1   tbsp. (15ml) chopped fresh thyme, divided
4   cloves garlic, minced
1   lemon, halved
1   medium onion, chopped and divided
6   medium carrots cut into 2-inch (5.08cm) pieces

1. Rinse chicken inside and out; pat dry with paper towels.
2. Rub 1 tablespoon (15ml) oil over chicken. Sprinkle chicken with 1 teaspoon (5ml) each of salt and pepper. Stir together 2 tablespoons (30ml) oil, 1½ teaspoons (7.5ml) thyme and garlic. Loosen skin from chicken, but do not totally detach. Rub oil mixture under skin. Place 1 lemon half and half of chopped onion into chicken. Squeeze remaining lemon into cavity.
3. Tie legs together; tuck wingtips under. Place chicken, breast side up, on greased rack in greased roasting pan.
4. Toss carrots and remaining onion with 2 tablespoons (30ml) olive oil, ½ teaspoon (2.5ml) salt, ½ teaspoon (2.5ml) pepper and 1½ teaspoons (7.5ml) thyme. Arrange carrot mixture in bottom of roasting pan.
5. Bake at 450°F (232°C) for 30 minutes. Reduce to 400°F (204°C) and bake 55 to 60 minutes or until a thermometer inserted into thigh registers 180°F (82°C). (Do not remove chicken from oven.) Cover with foil to prevent excessive browning.
6. Remove to a serving platter. Cover with foil and let stand 10 minutes before slicing. Arrange carrots and onions around chicken. Garnish with thyme sprigs and lemon slices, if desired.
Serves 6

Greek Leg of Lamb

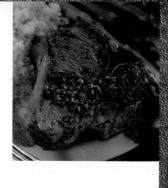

2 tbsp. (30ml) chopped fresh oregano
2 tbsp. (30ml) Greek seasoning
1½ tsp. (7.5ml) kosher salt
1 tsp. (5ml) cracked black pepper
2 cups (473ml) plain yogurt
3 tbsp. (44ml) olive oil
2 tbsp. (30ml) fresh lemon juice
1 (5- to 6-lb./2.3 to 2.7kg) leg of lamb, boned and trimmed

1. Whisk oregano, Greek seasoning, salt, pepper, yogurt, oil and lemon juice in a large bowl. Place lamb in a large shallow dish or heavy-duty resealable plastic bag. Pour yogurt mixture over lamb. Cover or seal, and refrigerate 2 hours, turning occasionally.
2. Remove lamb from marinade; discard marinade. Place lamb on a rack in a roasting pan.
3. Bake at 425°F (218°C) for 25 minutes; reduce temperature to 350°F (177°C) (do not remove meat from oven), and bake 1 hour and 15 minutes or until a meat thermometer inserted into thickest portion registers 145°F (63°C) for medium rare. Remove from oven and let stand 15 minutes or until a meat thermometer registers 150°F (66°C). Temperature will increase 5°F (2°C) upon standing.

Serves 8

Recipe Note: If preferred, marinate leg of lamb in yogurt mixture as long as overnight.

Lamb Chops with Cilantro Sauce

½ cup (118ml) fresh cilantro leaves
½ cup (118ml) mint leaves
2 tbsp. (30ml) honey
⅓ cup (79ml) rice wine vinegar
⅓ cup (79ml) plus 2 tbsp. (30ml) olive oil, divided
¼ tsp. (1ml) salt
½ tsp. (2.5ml) pepper
8 (4-oz./113g) lamb loin chops
Additional cilantro and mint leaves (optional)

1. In a food processor combine cilantro leaves, mint leaves, honey, vinegar, ⅓ cup (79ml) of the oil, salt and pepper; process until smooth. Pour ¼ cup (59ml) of the mixture over lamb chops in large shallow dish or resealable plastic bags; cover or seal and marinate in the refrigerator for 1 hour. Reserve remaining marinade mixture in the refrigerator.
2. Remove lamb chops from marinade; discard marinade. Heat the remaining 2 tablespoons (30ml) oil in a nonstick skillet over medium-high heat. Add lamb chops; cover and cook 13 minutes on each side or until meat thermometer registers 160°F (71°C).
3. Serve with reserved marinade and garnish with cilantro and mint leaves, if desired.

Serves 6

Lamb Burgers with Curried Mustard Sauce

1 egg, beaten
¼ cup (59ml) seasoned fine dry bread crumbs
1 lb. (454g) lean ground lamb
⅓ cup (79ml) light sour cream
1 tbsp. (15ml) Dijon mustard
½ tsp. (2.5ml) curry powder
8 slices French bread, toasted
Lettuce leaves and tomato slices (optional)

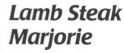

1. In a large bowl combine egg and bread crumbs. Add lamb; mix well. Shape lamb mixture into four ¾-inch-thick (1.9cm) patties.
2. Preheat grill to medium. Grill burgers, uncovered, for 14 to 18 minutes or until meat is done (170°F/77°C), turning once.
3. Meanwhile, for sauce combine sour cream, mustard and curry powder. Serve burgers on toasted bread with sauce. Add lettuce leaves and tomato slices, if desired.

Serves 4

Lamb Steak Marjorie

2 (6-oz./170g) lamb steaks, bone-in
2 cloves garlic
1 tbsp. (15ml) olive oil
2 drops hot pepper sauce
1 tsp. (5ml) dried marjoram (3 fresh leaves)

1. Trim visible fat from lamb.
2. Crush garlic and soak in oil and hot pepper sauce for 1 hour.
3. Brush steak with oil mixture; sprinkle with marjoram. Place in a resealable plastic bag and refrigerate for several hours or overnight.
4. Scrape off marjoram. Discard marinade. Broil steakes about 6 minutes per side (145°F/63°C) for medium rare.

Serves 2

Greek Pita Sandwich

- ½ lb. (227g) lean boneless lamb cutlet
- ¼ cup (59ml) plain low-fat yogurt
- 2 tbsp. (30ml) low-fat mayonnaise or salad dressing
- 1 tsp. (5ml) dried dill
- 1 clove garlic
- ¼ tsp. (1ml) onion powder
- 1 small cucumber, thinly sliced
- 1 small tomato, thinly sliced
- Pita bread

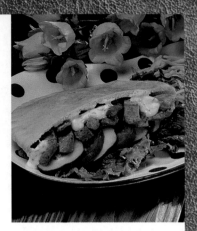

1. Slice lamb thinly across grain into bite-size strips.
2. Wrap pita in foil and heat in oven for 10 minutes at 350°F (177°C).
3. In small bowl combine yogurt, mayonnaise or salad dressing and dill. Set aside.
4. Spray or coat skillet or wok and preheat over medium-high heat. Add lamb, garlic and onion powder, stir-fry for 3 minutes or until meat is done and tender. Salt and pepper to taste.
5. Spread yogurt mixture inside warm pitas. Fill with meat, cucumber and tomato.

Serves 4

Lamb Chops with Yogurt Sauce

- 8 lamb loin or rib chops, cut 1 inch (2.54cm) thick
- ½ cup (118ml) plain low-fat yogurt
- ½ cup (118ml) chopped tomato
- ⅓ cup (79ml) chopped apple
- 3 tbsp. (44ml) raisins
- 3 tbsp. (44ml) chopped green onions
- ¼ tsp. (1ml) ground cinnamon
- Hot cooked couscous

1. Preheat grill to medium. Season chops with salt and pepper.
2. Grill chops, uncovered, to desired doneness, turning once. Allow 12 to 14 minutes for medium rare (145°F/63°C) and 15 to 17 minutes for medium (160°F/71°C).
3. Meanwhile, for sauce stir together yogurt, tomato, apple, raisins, green onions and cinnamon. Season to taste with salt.
4. Serve chops with couscous and yogurt sauce.

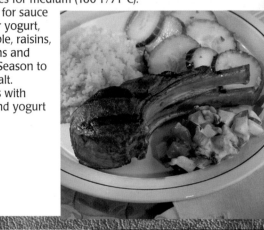

Serves 4

Lamb Chops with Apples and Thyme

- 8 lamb loin or rib chops, cut 1 inch (2.54cm) thick
- 1 tbsp. (15ml) olive oil
- 1 tbsp. (15ml) chopped fresh thyme leaves
- 1 clove garlic, minced
- 2 medium-tart cooking apples, cored and cut into 1-inch (2.54cm) slices
- 1 medium red onion, sliced ½ inch (1.27cm) thick

1. Preheat grill to medium.
2. Trim fat from chops. Combine olive oil, thyme and garlic. Brush oil mixture on both sides of chops and apple and onion slices.
3. Grill chops and apple and onion slices until chops are desired doneness and apples and onion are tender. (Allow 10 to 14 minutes for medium rare and 14 to 16 minutes for medium.)
4. Serve apple and onion rings with chops.

Serves 4

Savory Rack of Lamb

- 2 (1¼- to 1 ½-lb./567 to 680g) lamb rib roasts (6 to 8 ribs each)
- 4 cloves garlic, minced
- 1 tbsp. (15ml) chopped fresh rosemary or 2 tsp. (10ml) dried rosemary
- 1 tsp. (5ml) olive oil
- ½ tsp. (2.5ml) finely shredded lemon peel
- ½ tsp. (2.5ml) salt
- Freshly ground black pepper

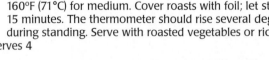

1. Preheat oven to 325°F (163°C). Trim excess fat from roasts, if necessary. Combine garlic, rosemary, olive oil, lemon peel and salt. Rub over meat. Place roasts bone side down on a rack in a shallow roasting pan. Sprinkle with pepper. Insert meat thermometer in thickest part of roast, being sure it is not touching bone.
2. Roast, uncovered, for 45 minutes to 1 hour or until meat thermometer registers 140°F (60°C) for medium rare, 160°F (71°C) for medium. Cover roasts with foil; let stand 15 minutes. The thermometer should rise several degrees during standing. Serve with roasted vegetables or rice pilaf.

Serves 4

Red Snapper Baked in Wine

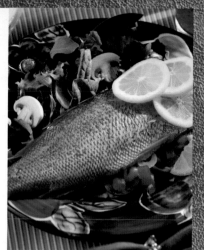

- 1 (3-lb./1.36kg) fresh or thawed dressed whole red snapper
- 1 medium onion, thinly sliced
- 1 medium green bell pepper, thinly sliced
- 1 medium tomato, chopped
- 1 tsp. (5ml) dried thyme, crushed
- 1 tbsp. (15ml) olive oil
- ⅓ cup (79ml) dry white wine
- Lemon wedges (optional)

1. Preheat oven to 400°F (204°C). Rinse fish; pat dry with paper towels. Layer onion, pepper and tomato in cavity of fish. Sprinkle with thyme.
2. Line 15x10x1-inch (25x38x2.5-cm) jelly-roll pan with foil. Place fish in pan. Brush with some oil. Drizzle wine over fish.
3. Bake for 15 minutes. Turn fish. Brush with remaining oil. Bake for 15 to 25 minutes more or until fish begins to flake with a fork (145°F/63°C). Serve with lemon wedges, if desired.

Serves 6

Shrimp Paella

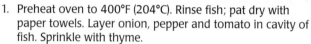

- 1 (14½-oz./411g) can diced tomatoes
- 1 (6¾-oz./191g) pkg. regular Spanish-style rice mix
- 8 oz. (227g) fresh or thawed shrimp, peeled and deveined
- 4 cups (.95l) sliced yellow onions
- 1 green bell pepper, sliced
- 2 tbsp. (30ml) olive oil
- 8 cloves garlic, minced
- 2 cups (473ml) thawed peas
- 1 tbsp. (15ml) lemon juice

1. In a medium saucepan prepare undrained tomatoes and rice mix according to rice package directions.
2. Meanwhile, rinse shrimp; pat dry with paper towels. In a 12-inch (30.5cm) skillet cook onions and pepper in hot oil over medium heat until tender, stirring frequently. Stir in shrimp and garlic. Cook and stir for 3 to 4 minutes or until shrimp turn opaque.
3. Stir hot rice mixture, peas and lemon juice into shrimp mixture.

Serves 4

Grilled Lemon-Butter Lobster

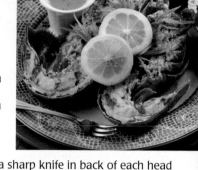

- 2 (1¼- to 1½-lb./567 to 680g) live lobsters
- ¼ cup (59ml) butter or margarine
- 2 tbsp. (30ml) lemon juice
- 1 tbsp. (15ml) finely shredded lemon peel
- 2 tsp. (10ml) chopped fresh tarragon
- 2 tsp. (10ml) chopped fresh chives
- ¾ cup (178ml) fresh bread crumbs (1 slice)

1. Kill lobsters by inserting a sharp knife in back of each head between eyes. Use kitchen scissors to make 2 cuts lengthwise and crosswise in underside of. Remove membrane. Open tails. Scrape out black vein. Remove and discard organs near head. Rinse. Pat dry with paper towels.
2. Lightly coat the grill rack with nonstick cooking spray. Preheat the grill to medium. Prepare grill for indirect cooking.
3. In a small saucepan cook and stir butter, lemon juice, lemon peel, tarragon and chives over low heat until butter is melted.
4. Place lobsters, shell-side down, on the grill rack. Brush with some butter mixture. Grill, covered, for 20 to 30 minutes or until meat is nearly opaque, brushing twice with butter mixture. Do not turn. Sprinkle with bread crumbs and drizzle with remaining butter mixture. Cover and grill for 10 to 12 minutes more or until meat is opaque.

Serves 2

Cucumber-Topped Cod

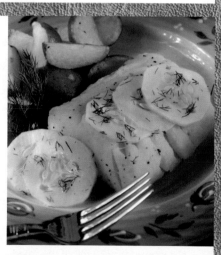

- 2 (6-oz./170g) fresh or thawed cod fillets, about ½ inch (1.27cm) thick
- ¼ cup (58ml) flour
- 2 tbsp. (30ml) butter or margarine
- 1 cup (237ml) peeled and sliced cucumber
- 1 clove garlic, minced
- 1 tsp. (5ml) chopped fresh dill weed
- 1 tbsp. (15ml) lemon juice

1. Rinse fish; pat dry with paper towels. Coat fish with flour. Season with salt and pepper.
2. In a large skillet heat butter. Add fish. Cook over medium heat for 5 to 6 minutes or until fish flakes with a fork (145°F/63°C), turning once. Transfer to a warm platter.
3. Add cucumber, garlic and dill to skillet. Cook for 2 minutes. Add lemon juice. Cook 1 minute more. Spoon over cod.

Serves 2

Honey Mustard Scallop Kabobs

1   lb. (454g) sea scallops
2   tbsp. (30ml) honey
2   tbsp. (30ml) cooking oil
1   tbsp. (15ml) country Dijon mustard
2   tsp. (10ml) Worcestershire sauce
1   cup (237ml) fresh or canned pineapple chunks
1   medium green bell pepper, cut into 16 pieces

1. Place scallops in a resealable plastic bag. Combine honey, oil, mustard and Worcestershire sauce. Set aside 1 tablespoon (15ml) of mixture in the refrigerator. Pour remaining honey mixture over scallops. Seal bag and refrigerate 30 minutes.
2. Preheat grill to medium. Drain scallops; discard marinade. Alternately thread scallops, pineapple and green pepper onto 8 metal skewers.
3. Grill for 5 to 8 minutes, turning once, or until scallops are opaque. Brush with reserved honey mixture just before removing from grill.

Serves 4

Baked Fish with Vegetables

1   lb. (454g) fresh or frozen salmon or other fish fillets, ½ to ¾ inch (1.27 to 1.9cm) thick
2   small zucchini, cut into ¼-inch (.64cm) slices (2 cups/473ml)
1   medium green bell pepper, cut into thin strips (1 cup/237ml)
1   medium onion, thinly sliced
1   tbsp. (15ml) vegetable oil
2   small plum tomatoes, chopped (½ cup/118ml)
1   tbsp. (15ml) juice from a fresh lemon
½   tsp. (2.5ml) basil leaves
¼   tsp. (1ml) coarse ground black pepper
Dash bottled hot pepper sauce
¼ cup (59ml) shredded Parmesan cheese

1. Thaw fish, if frozen. Preheat oven to 450°F (232°C). Lightly coat a 2-quart (2l) square baking dish with nonstick cooking spray. Cut fish into serving-size pieces and arrange in prepared dish.
2. In a large skillet cook zucchini, green pepper and onion in hot oil for 2 to 3 minutes or until crisp-tender. Spoon over fish. Top with tomatoes.
3. Stir together lemon juice, ½ teaspoon (2.5ml) salt, basil, pepper and hot pepper sauce. Sprinkle over fish and vegetables.
4. Bake, uncovered, for 12 to 18 minutes or until fish flakes easily with a fork. Transfer fish and vegetables to a serving plate. Sprinkle with cheese.

Serves 4

Grilled Tuna Nicoise salad

1¼ lb. (567g) fresh or thawed tuna steaks, about 1 inch (2.5cm) thick
3   Roma tomatoes, halved lengthwise
8   oz. (227g) asparagus spears, trimmed
2   tbsp. (30ml) bottled Caesar salad dressing
8   cups (2l) assorted torn greens
2   hard-cooked eggs, chopped or sliced
⅓   cup (79ml) pitted Nicoise olives or ripe olives
¾   cup (178ml) bottled Caesar salad dressing

1. Lightly coat the grill rack with nonstick cooking spray. Preheat the grill to medium.
2. Rinse fish; pat dry with paper towels. Cut into 6 serving-size pieces. Brush tuna steaks, tomato halves, and asparagus with 2 tablespoons (30 ml) of the salad dressing.
3. Grill tuna for 10 to 12 minutes or until fish flakes with a fork (145°F/63°C), turning once. Place tomato halves and asparagus on the grill 7 minutes after starting tuna, cooking for 3 to 4 minutes or until tomatoes are heated through and asparagus is tender.
4. Divide greens among 6 dinner plates. Arrange grilled tuna, tomatoes and asparagus on top of greens. Sprinkle with hard-cooked egg and olives. Drizzle with remaining ¾ cup (178 ml) salad dressing.

Serves 6

Crab-Cheese Wontons

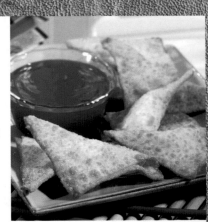

1   tub (12 oz./340g) soft cream cheese spread
¼   cup (59ml) crabmeat, finely chopped (canned or fresh)
¼   tsp. (1ml) garlic salt
1   (16 oz./454g) pkg. wonton wrappers
Vegetable oil
Purchased sweet and sour sauce or plum sauce (optional)

1. In bowl stir together cream cheese spread, crabmeat and garlic salt. Place about 1 teaspoon (5ml) in center of each wonton wrapper square. Moisten edges lightly with water. Fold squares in half, bringing 2 opposite corners together forming a triangle. Press edges to seal.
2. In skillet heat about ¾ inch (1.9cm) of vegetable oil over medium-high heat to about 325°F (163°C). Fry several wontons at a time for 3 to 4 minutes or until golden, turning once. Drain on paper towels. If desired, serve with sweet and sour sauce or plum sauce.

Makes 45

glossary of cooking terms

BAKING	To cook food in an oven at a specified temperature.
BARBECUING	A method of long, slow cooking in a pit, on a spit or in a kettle grill over indirect heat.
BRAISING	A method of moist cooking. The meat is browned on both sides in a small amount of oil to seal in the juices. Liquid is added and the meat is cooked, tightly covered, over low heat for a long time to tenderize it.
BROIL	To cook with the heat source above the meat. If using an electric oven, leave the door ajar or the thermostat will turn off the broiler at 500°F (260°C). Meat should be turned once to cook both sides.
DEEP-FRYING	To cook food by submerging it in deep, hot oil.
DEGREASING	To skim fat from the surface of a hot liquid. If chilled, the fat will rise to the surface and become solid, making it easy to remove.
DONENESS	There are 4 degrees of doneness for meat: rare, medium rare, medium and well done. They vary for each variety of meat. Check the individual charts.
DREDGING	To lightly coat meat or fowl with flour or cornmeal before cooking.
GRILLING	To cook with a heat source from below in the form of gas or charcoal. Covered grills allow you to slow-roast large pieces of meat and poultry over indirect heat (the coals are pushed to one side and the meat is on the other).
MARINATING	Marinades are used to improve the flavor and tenderize less expensive cuts of meat. Seafood can actually "cook" in citrus-based marinades without heat. Be sure to discard any unused marinade after initial use.
PAN-BROILING	To cook meat in a heavy pan with little or no fat over medium-high heat. Fat and juices are poured off as they appear.
PAN-FRYING	To cook food in a small amount of hot oil over medium-high heat.
POACHING	To gently cook food in a liquid that is hot, but not boiling.
OVEN-ROASTING	Roasting and baking are the same form of dry-heat cooking.
SAUTÉING	To cook food in a small amount of hot oil over medium-high heat. It is similar to pan-frying, but less oil is used.
SEARING	To brown meat with intense heat in order to seal in the juices.
SMOKING	To slowly cook food over low heat (below 180°F or 82°C) for a long period. Usually, some liquid is added to provide smoke. True smoking is not safe for the home cook. Bacteria grows rapidly below 200°F (93°C). A similar flavor can be achieved safely with mini-barbecue pits.
STEAMING	To cook food on a rack above steaming water in a covered pot.
STIR-FRYING	To cook bite-size pieces in a small amount of oil over high heat.

glossary of general meat terms

AGING	Aging causes an enzyme change that deepens the flavor and color of meat. The longer meat is aged, the quicker it will cook.
DRY AGED and FAST AGED	Dry aged meat is kept at 34°F to 38°F (1°C to 3°C) for 10 days to 6 weeks. Fast aged meat is held at 70°F (21°C) for 2 days with controlled humidity. Ultraviolet lights reduce the chance of bacterial growth.
FREEZER BURN	This occurs when meat has been improperly wrapped, or kept too long in the freezer. The meat loses moisture, leaving a dry, grayish surface. Freezer burn affects both the taste and the texture.
GRADE	A method of judging meat quality. It is not the same as meat inspection. The United States Department of Agriculture, the department of Agriculture and Agri-Food Canada, the manufacturer or the retailer determines grades. Grading is voluntary, except where local laws require it.
HIGH QUALITY	A grade of meat. High quality beef comes from animals with broad and substantial backs. The more loin available, the better the quality.
MARBLING	The "tasty" fat that gives meat its juicy tenderness and flavor. It appears as flecks or strands in the meat. It cannot be trimmed.
MEAT INSPECTION	The United States Department of Agriculture (USDA) and Agriculture and Agri-Food Canada (AAFC) are responsible for assuring the safety and quality of foods. They conduct inspections for sanitation and cleanliness, labeling and packing at facilities where meat and poultry are cut up, boned, cured and canned to ensure the safety of their nation's meat.
MOLLUSKS	Soft-bodied and often hard-shelled animals, including snails, clams, oysters, mussells, scallops, octopus and squid.
OMEGA-3	A special type of polyunsaturated fat found in seafood that helps lower cholesterol levels, as well as provide other health benefits.
OFFAL	Another name for organ meats, such as brains, stomach (tripe), kidneys, sweetmeats, liver and tongue.
PRAWN	A term used to describe very large shrimp. It is also the name for crustaceans resembling small lobsters and fresh water shrimp.
PROCESSED MEAT	Meats that have been changed by cooking, curing, drying or canning.
RED MEAT	The result of heavily worked muscles that hold more oxygen, which gives the meat a red color. Chickens are flightless birds, so their breasts are not red, but their legs, which they use, are "dark meat."
VACUUM PACKING	A method of reducing moisture loss in packaged meats. By removing all the air from the package, the meat will last longer. The color of the meat will appear to be somewhat purplish, but will change when exposed to air.
WHITE MEAT	Refers to animal muscles, or meat, which is pale. A meat's color is determined by the amount of exercise it does. If the muscle is heavily worked, it will hold more oxygen. Oxygen is what makes meat dark.